Practical Handbook of
FLUORESCEIN
ANGIOGRAPHY

D1614013

Practical Handbook of
FLUORESCEIN ANGIOGRAPHY

Bruno Lumbroso

Rome, Italy

Marco Rispoli

Rome, Italy

Library Resource Center
Renton Technical College
3000 N.E. 4th Street
Renton, USA 98056

JAYPEE BROTHERS MEDICAL PUBLISHERS (P) LTD

New Delhi • London • Philadelphia • Panama

Jaypee Brothers Medical Publishers (P) Ltd

Headquarters

Jaypee Brothers Medical Publishers (P) Ltd
4838/24, Ansari Road, Daryaganj
New Delhi 110 002, India
Phone: +91-11-43574357
Fax: +91-11-43574314
Email: jaypee@jaypeebrothers.com

Overseas Offices

J.P. Medical Ltd
83 Victoria Street, London
SW1H 0HW (UK)
Phone: +44-2031708910
Fax: +02-03-0086180
Email: info@jpmedpub.com

Jaypee Medical Inc.
The Bourse
111 South Independence Mall East
Suite 835, Philadelphia, PA 19106, USA
Phone: + 267-519-9789
Email: joe.rusko@jaypeebrothers.com

Jaypee Brothers Medical Publishers (P) Ltd
Bhotahity, Kathmandu, Nepal
Phone: +977-9741283608
Email: kathmandu@jaypeebrothers.com

Jaypee-Highlights Medical Publishers Inc.
City of Knowledge, Bld. 237, Clayton
Panama City, Panama
Phone: + 507-301-0496
Fax: + 507-301-0499
Email: cservice@jphmedical.com

Jaypee Brothers Medical Publishers (P) Ltd
17/1-B Babar Road, Block-B, Shaymali
Mohammadpur, Dhaka-1207
Bangladesh
Mobile: +08801912003485
Email: jaypeedhaka@gmail.com

Website: www.jaypeebrothers.com
Website: www.jaypeedigital.com

© 2014, Jaypee Brothers Medical Publishers

The views and opinions expressed in this book are solely those of the original contributor(s)/author(s) and do not necessarily represent those of editor(s) of the book.

All rights reserved. No part of this publication may be reproduced, stored or transmitted in any form or by any means, electronic, mechanical, photocopying, recording or otherwise, without the prior permission in writing of the publishers.

All brand names and product names used in this book are trade names, service marks, trademarks or registered trademarks of their respective owners. The publisher is not associated with any product or vendor mentioned in this book.

Medical knowledge and practice change constantly. This book is designed to provide accurate, authoritative information about the subject matter in question. However, readers are advised to check the most current information available on procedures included and check information from the manufacturer of each product to be administered, to verify the recommended dose, formula, method and duration of administration, adverse effects and contraindications. It is the responsibility of the practitioner to take all appropriate safety precautions. Neither the publisher nor the author(s)/editor(s) assume any liability for any injury and/or damage to persons or property arising from or related to use of material in this book.

This book is sold on the understanding that the publisher is not engaged in providing professional medical services. If such advice or services are required, the services of a competent medical professional should be sought.

Every effort has been made where necessary to contact holders of copyright to obtain permission to reproduce copyright material. If any have been inadvertently overlooked, the publisher will be pleased to make the necessary arrangements at the first opportunity.

Inquiries for bulk sales may be solicited at: jaypee@jaypeebrothers.com

Practical Handbook of Fluorescein Angiography

First Edition: **2014**

ISBN: 978-93-5090-991-1

Printed at Replika Press Pvt. Ltd.

617.730754 LUMBROS 2014

Lumbroso, Bruno,

Practical handbook of
fluorescein angiography

Preface

I (Bruno Lumbroso) have been teaching for years logical methods of retinal imaging analysis and interpretation. I published my first *Handbook of Fluorescein Angiography Interpretation* a few years after the fluorescein angiography clinical use became widespread. After it, I published analytical manuals on indocyanine green angiography and, lately, OCT (cross section and "en face" OCT).

In these interpretation handbooks, I systematically follow a rational method to interpret medical ophthalmological imaging. Accurate analysis must come before synthesis deduction and diagnosis. Diagnoses must be the product of logical processes. The inability to formulate an exact diagnosis could be due to the insufficient logical exploitation of one's knowledge.

Even now, with the extensive use of OCT, Fluorescein Angiography remains absolutely necessary in clinical ophthalmology to detect and highlight retinal alterations in morphology and structure.

Widely illustrated with Fluorescein Angiography figures but also, when necessary with ICG, Autofluorescence, sagittal and frontal OCT images, this concise handbook intends to show how to read and interpret Fluorescein Angiography imaging, documenting and diagnosing the most common retinal pathologies. Several tables not only offer guidance through everyday disorders but also in the difficult study of the rarest and most difficult diagnoses. This manual illustrates a logical and simple analysis and interpretation method of Fluorescein Angiography imaging, clearly stating the steps required to reach a diagnosis.

I am happy today to propose this new Practical Handbook of Fluorescein Angiography, not only to young doctors and residents but also to ophthalmologists more expert with retinal diseases.

I (Bruno Lumbroso) would like to thank Dr Marco Rispoli for his many years of invaluable collaboration, unerring imaging and image selection, and help with the chapters of this volume.

Bruno Lumbroso
Marco Rispoli

Contents

Part III: Pathological Fluorescein Angiography Analytical Study

PART I

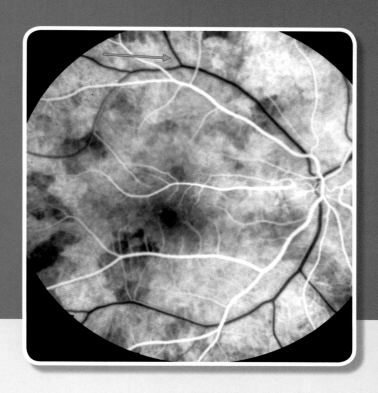

Interpretation

Retinal Anatomy and Fluorescein Angiography

The analytical study of retinal anatomy in relation to fluorescence angiography requires the retina to be subdivided into the *posterior pole* that lies inside the vascular arcades, and the *peripheral retina* that is the area around the posterior pole and the optic disc. The peripheral retina is further divided into nasal periphery and upper and lower temporal periphery.

POSTERIOR POLE

The longer horizontal axis of the oval-shaped *posterior pole* measures 8–10 millimeters (30–35°). Fluorescein angiography with a 45° angle allows for a single frame picture to be taken of the posterior pole, the optic disc and part of the vascular arcades. Modern devices allow wide angle angiography.

MACULAR AREA

The *macula*, with a thickness of 100 microns, is located at the center of the posterior pole where it forms a slight depression centered on the fovea and the foveola. It has a 1200-micron diameter. Within the macular area fluorescein angiography we observe the *avascular* area that has a diameter of 450–500 microns and is sharply highlighted by the dye in the capillary phase. This dark avascular area is delimited by a continuous ring of fine anastomoses of the perifoveal vascular network, consisting of a single layer of capillaries.

The fovea itself, which is anatomically an area with a larger concentration of cones, is contained within a concentric circle having a diameter of 350 microns, hence it lies inside the fluorescein angiographic avascular area, while the foveola, that corresponds to the macular center, measures about 100 microns. In the macula, there is a strong density of xanthophyllic pigment and at this level the cells of the pigment epithelium are higher and contain a bigger density of pigment granules. Apart from the absence of rods, the other specific feature of the macula is the decreased thickness of the retina, and the thickening of the inner nuclear layers at the macula margins.

Around the macula area, the retina is 350 microns thick. Let us recall the nine layers of the retina: from the inner layer towards the outer layer we find the internal limiting membrane, the nerve fibers layer, ganglion cells layer, inner plexiform layer, inner nuclear layer (bipolar cells bodies), outer plexiform layer, outer nuclear layer (cones and rods cellular bodies), outer limiting membrane, cones and rods layer. Then there is the external retinal layer consisting of a single layer of pigmented epithelial cells in close contact with each other through their "tight junctions". These pigment epithelium cells are linked to each other and to Bruch's membrane or to the lamina vitrea by a cementing substance. The lamina vitrea is part of the choroid that is divided into choriocapillaris and choroid proper.

RETINAL ARTERIES AND VEINS

The optic disc has a diameter of 1500 microns whereas the retinal veins at the border of the disc have a maximum diameter of about 120 microns. At the mid-periphery, their diameter is about 60 microns. The retinal arteries have a slightly smaller diameter (respectively 80 and 50 microns). The capillaries in immediate contact with the retinal vessels are very scarce and virtually absent (periarterial avascular area). At the arteriovenous crossings, arteries and veins are united by a common adventitia. The size of retinal capillaries ranges between 5 and 10 microns.

The sensory retina is supplied by two separate vascular systems. The inner side is supplied by retinal vessels; the most important branches are located in the nerve fiber level and form a loose network whereas the capillaries are observed in the inner half of the retina up to the inner nuclear layer and form a closer-knit network. The outer third of the retina instead is supplied by the choroid vascular system.

THE CHOROID

The choroid is part of the vascular tunica of the eye and consists of dense vascular tissue where the larger vessels are positioned externally, close to the sclera (Haller layer), the smaller vessels are in the inner part (Sattler layer), and the choriocapillaris is in contact with the retina.

The choroid is supplied by the posterior ciliary arteries (about 15–20 branches). The vascular supply to the choroid is schematized in Figure 1 that indicates the districts supplied by each branch of the short and long posterior ciliary arteries. The districts are clearly separated from each other and form distinct wedges or triangles (Fig. 1).

This figure helps understand the fluorescein angiographic aspect of certain occlusive lesions of the choroid (triangular syndromes). The most important vessels are impermeable to fluorescein and are in contact with the sclera. They are visible on the fluorescein angiography in the presence of sclerosis of the choriocapillaris and of the retinal pigment epithelium (window lesions). The arteries subdivide rapidly forming *lobules*, small, irregular, distinct independent and not inter-linked units. Each unit or lobule is functionally independent from the others. The lobule measures about 250 × 300 microns. All the lobules together form the choriocapillaris whose capillaries are larger in size than other capillaries (20 microns) and they have fenestrated walls that allow the fluorescein to rapidly diffuse. The choriocapillaris provides nutrition and oxygen to the outer third of the retina (pigment epithelium, cones and rods).

The veins of the choroid, originating from each lobule, flow into the 4 or 6 vortex veins located in the four quadrants of the bulb at the equator.

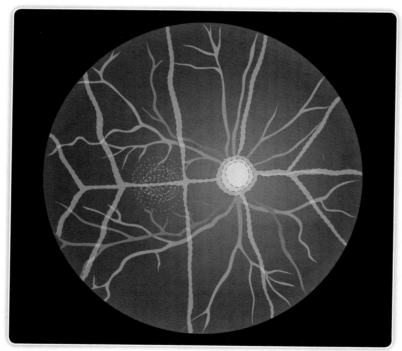

Figure 1: Choroid Vascular Supply. Choroid is supplied by the posterior ciliary arteries (from Hayreh, modified)—vascular districts form distinct wedges or triangle.

Normal Fluorescein Angiography of the Retina

This chapter describes fluorescein angiography from the clinical standpoint without insisting on the more specifically technical or anatomic aspects. Practically a normal fluorescein angiography can be divided, as shown in Table 1, into 7 phases: arm retina phase, choroidal phase, arterial phase, capillary phase or arterial-venous phase, early venous phase, late venous phase, tissue phase.

ARM TO RETINA PHASE

After injecting the fluorescein bolus into the vein of the elbow, the fluorescein penetrates into the retinal vessels after about 10–12 seconds in a normal individual. This phase may however vary in dependence of the cardiovascular conditions of the patient, blood viscosity, and size of the blood vessels that influence the circulation rate. It is important to compare the phases of the arm to retina phase of the two sides: we could so highlight any alterations in the carotid circulation.

CHOROIDAL PHASE

By penetrating through the short ciliary vessels, the fluorescein will initially highlight irregularly the vessels of the choriocapillaris, like a geographic map. In normal patients this phase varies considerably from individual to individual. During the choroidal phase the ciliary-retinal arteries (retinal arteries that originate directly from the choroid), when present, will be filled and stand out very clearly against a gray background because the remaining retinal vessels have not yet been reached (Fig. 7). In any case, it is always very difficult to study the choroidal circulation because the pigment epithelium acts as a screen and prevents it from standing out and above all the rapid diffusion of the dye through the vessels of the choriocapillaris in the subsequent phases, makes the choroid almost evenly fluorescent, with very slight variations (Figs 1 and 2).

ARTERIAL PHASE

The central artery of the retina and its branches fill rapidly. The filling occurs homogeneously throughout the arterial vessel and its branches. Often there are variations in the time it takes the arterial branches to fill; the nasal arteries generally fill later than the temporal arteries. The differences from individual to individual are however quite sizeable.

	Table 1: Normal fluorescein angiography	
	Arm retina phase	About 10–12 seconds
10–12 sec	Choroidal phase	Geographic map-like filling of the choroid. Filling of the ciliary-retinal arteries
11–14 sec	Arterial phase	Filling of the central retinal artery and of its ramifications. The filling of the choroid is completed
12–15 sec	Capillary or arterial-venous phase	Visualization of the capillary network of the posterior pole
13–16 sec	Early venous phase	Initial laminar filling of the veins
15–20 sec	Venous phase	Progressive filling of the venous lumen
1–10 min	Tissue time (very late phase)	Progressive reduction of the vascular fluorescence. Persistence of a slight fluorescence due to staining of the optic disc and of the choroid

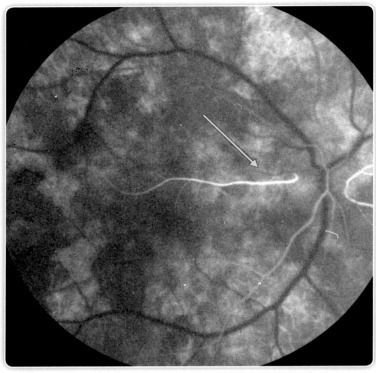

Figure 1: Choroidal Phase 1. A light blush is observed. A ciliary artery fills before the other retinal arteries.

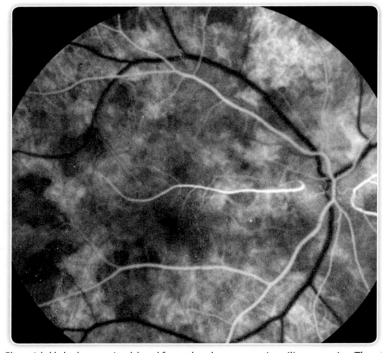

Figure 2: Choroidal Phase 2. Choroidal lobules receive blood from the short posterior ciliary arteries. They fill irregularly, giving a checker appearance to the angiograph.

THE CAPILLARY OR ARTERIO-VENOUS PHASE

The capillary phase is very brief but especially in younger individuals beautiful pictures can be obtained that highlight in particular, the perifoveal network that is clearly visible against the hyperpigmented background of the macular region. It is much more difficult to show up the radial capillary network starting from the papilla. The macula is normally always darker for three reasons: 1) presence of xanthophyllic pigment, 2) greater pigmentation of the cells of the pigment epithelium that hide the normal fluorescence of the choroid and, 3) absence of capillaries in the avascular region of the fovea. When the capillary network of the macular is too evident, it is very likely pathological, dilated and with interrupted web. Note also the beginning of the venous laminar flow (Fig. 3).

VENOUS PHASE

The peculiar characteristic of the venous phase is the filling of the veins through laminar flow. This means that the fluorescein penetrates first of all along the walls of the veins. It is a cylindrical filling in which the peripheral blood penetrates into the veins at a later stage when it then occupies the central part of the lumen (Figs 6A and B).

This early *venous phase* begins normally 5 or 6 seconds after the choroidal phase. From each supplying vein the laminar flow can be noticed; it preserves its autonomy for a certain time even in the larger branches where at times several concentric laminae of fluorescein can be noticed that show the topographic origin of the venous blood until the main vascular trunk. The venous phase lasts about 2-3 seconds during which the veins fill completely and they show the highest possible fluorescence.

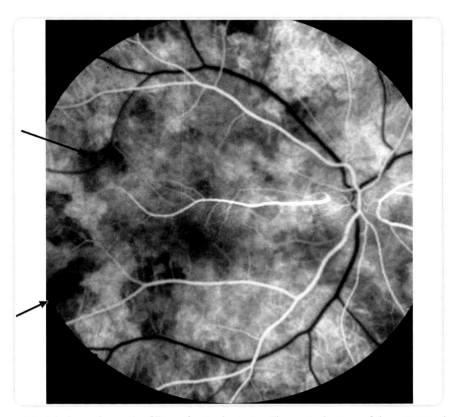

Figure 3: Arterial Phase. Arterial phase shows the filling of retinal arteries. The central artery of the retina and its branches fill rapidly. Filling occurs homogeneously throughout the central artery and its branches. Some choroidal lobules are not yet filled (arrows).

Then the fluorescence of the venous vessels begins to decrease slowly thus constituting the *late venous* phase. The less fluorescent aspect of these phases may to some extent also be due to the fact that the choroid gets completely stained by the fluorescein and therefore there is less contrast between the fluorescein present in the vessels and the fluorescence of the fundus of the eye (Figs 4A and B and 6A and B).

TISSUE PHASE

From 5–10 minutes after the injection of the fluorescein there is hardly ever any normal fluorescence in the tissues, except the optic disc. Any fluorescence that can be observed is due to pathologic conditions that are to be observed very carefully in order to interpret the retinal or choroidal alterations. This issue will be discussed in depth in the chapter on the interpretation of pathological fluorescein angiographies (Fig. 5).

PSEUDOFLUORESCENCE

When the two filters of the retinograph, blue excitation and green, have transmission curves that partly overlap, they are not totally dye-proof. In this case, the light reflected from structures of the fundus may seep through and impress the photographic film, thus producing a pseudofluorescence. With the current fluorescein angiography devices, endowed with interference filters, this phenomenon hardly ever occurs.

AUTOFLUORESCENCE

Some pathological structures of the fundus (drusen of the papilla, astrocytic hamartomas) have the property of spontaneously producing fluorescent light when they are stimulated by blue light. Retinal Pigment epithelium autofluorescence is due to the presence of lipofuscin—in vivo autofluorescence clinical study is recent.

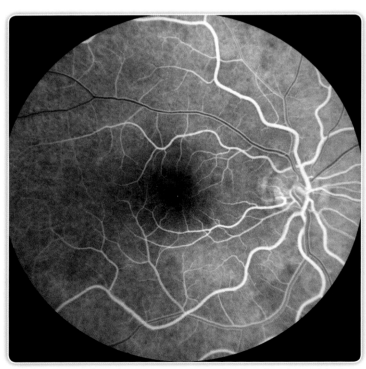

Figure 4A: Early Venous Phase. Early venous phase begins 5 or 6 seconds after the choroidal phase. From each supplying vein the laminar flow coming from peripheral retina can be noticed; the laminar flow preserves its independence and individuality for a certain time even in the larger branches where at times several concentric laminae of fluorescein can be noticed that reveal the topographic origin of the venous blood in the vascular main trunk. Some choroidal lobules are not yet filled.

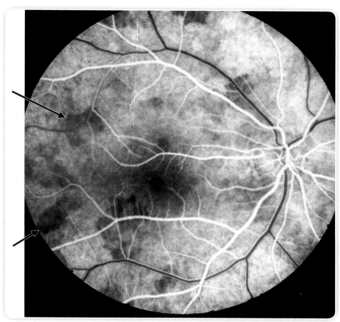

Figure 4B: Late Venous Phase. Late venous phase begins 2 seconds after the early phase. Each vein is fully filled and shows an even flow. Then fluorescence of the venous vessels decreases slowly thus constituting the late venous phase. The less fluorescent aspect of these phases may to some extent also be due to the fact that the choroid gets fully stained by the fluorescein and therefore there is less contrast between the fluorescein present in the vessels and the fluorescence of the fundus of the eye. Arrows indicate choroid territories not yet filled.

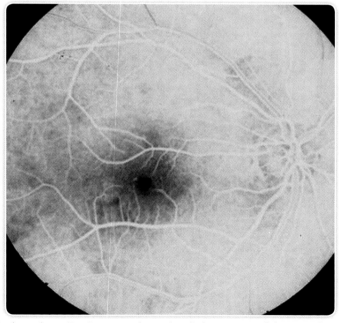

Figure 5: Late Tissue Phase. In the late phase (3 minutes and more) a slight staining of the retinal and optic disc can be seen. Later on, from 5–10 minutes after the injection of the fluorescein there is hardly ever any normal fluorescence in the tissues, except the optic disc. Any fluorescence is due to pathologic conditions that are to be observed very carefully in order to interpret the retinal or choroidal alterations.

Checking for the presence of such autofluorescence by taking photographs before injecting the fluorescein may be useful to distinguish a papillary pseudoedema caused by drusen from a true papillary edema. With modern angiography devices autofluorescence study has greatly developed. Autofluorescence imaging is now widely used for diagnosis in patients with visual loss and in inherited maculopathy.

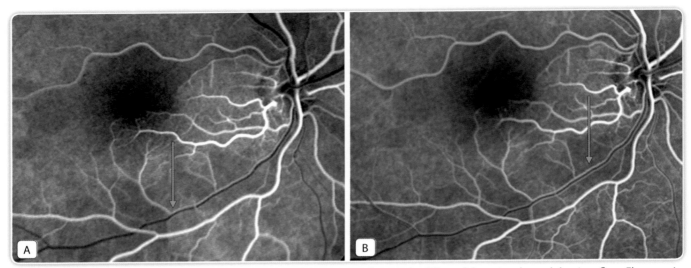

Figures 6A and B: Laminar Flow. An interesting feature of the venous phase is the filling of the veins through laminar flow. Fluorescein enters the vessels first of all along the walls of the veins. It forms a cylinder along the walls (arrow). Later the peripheral blood penetrates into the vein center.

A.   Early venous phase begins normally 5 or 6 seconds after the choroidal phase. From each supplying vein the laminar flow can be noticed; it preserves its autonomy for a certain time even in the larger branches where at times several concentric laminae of fluorescein can be noticed that show the topographic origin of the venous blood also in the vascular trunk (arrow).

B.   Later venous phase. Venous lamellar filling is not yet completed.

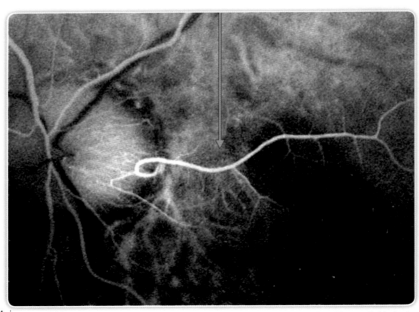

Figure 7: Ciliary Artery. A ciliary artery fills before the other retinal arteries (arrow). As the choroidal lobules it receives blood directly from the short posterior ciliary arteries. Some choroidal lobules are not yet filled.

CHAPTER 3

Normal Fluorescein Angiogram of the Optic Disc

The capillaries of the deep prelaminar network fill at the same time as the choroid and the cilio-retinal arteries. A second later, the fluorescence of the superficial capillary network supplied by the central retinal artery begins. These structures have a roughly radial aspect and they immediately mask the deeper capillaries.

This phase occurs simultaneously with the retinal arterial phase and is immediately followed by a diffused hyperfluorescence at the early and later venous phases that does not allow to identify the details of the vascular network of the optic disc. There are frequently parapapillary areas that are hyperfluorescent due to the local absence of pigment or they are hypofluorescent due to localized hyperpigmentation.

In the later phases, the optic disc presents a light diffuse hyperfluorescence that may last two or three hours, due to the staining of the deep structures and of the lamina cribrosa. This hyperfluorescence is even more persistent at the edges of the disc (Table 1) (Figs 1A to E).

Table 1: Normal optic disc	
• **Choroidal phase**	Filling of the deep prelaminar network (simultaneously with cilioretinal filling, if any)
• **Arterial phase**	Filling of the epipapillary radial network that hides the deeper vessels; increase in the fluorescence of the disc
• **Venous phase**	Venous details not very visible
• **Late phases** (tissue phase)	Diffused hyperfluorescence that decreases progressively and may persist on the disc edges for more than an hour
	• Possible areas of parapapillary hyperfluorescence due to depigmentation or hypofluorescence due to hyperpigmentation

Library Resource Center
Renton Technical College
3000 N.E. 4th Street
Renton, WA 98056

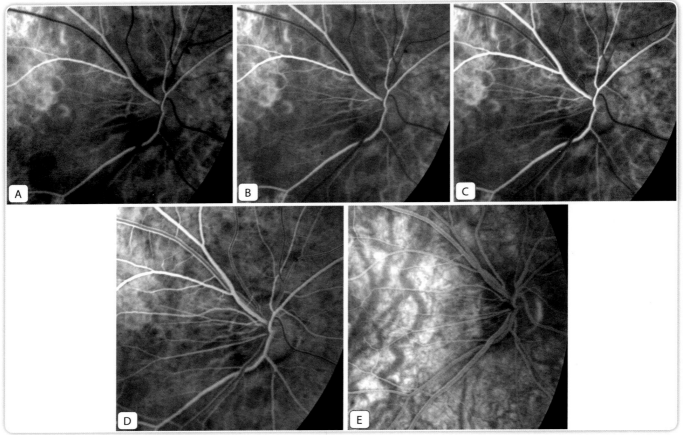

Figures 1A to E: The different phases of the optic disc filling are highlighted in the figures: (A) Choroidal phase; (B) Arterial filling; (C and D) Venous phase; (E) Late phase

CHAPTER 4

Normal Fluorescein Angiography of the Choroid

Choroid circulation is very difficult to highlight in normal conditions. Indeed it is usually masked when the pigment epithelium is normal. When it is visible, it is rapidly overshadowed by the staining of the retinal vascular tree. In the case of albino eyes, the early phases of the choroid fluorescein angiography provide a sharp picture.

Filling of the main choroid vessels occurs a second before the retinal arterial phase because the main choroid vessels are filled through the ciliary vessels. The main choroid vessels can be seen very rarely, even in the best cases. The vessels of the choriocapillaris fill in an irregular way giving the fundus the aspect of a geographic map (See Chapter 2 Figs 1 to 4A and B). This is due mainly to the slightly deferred filling of the lobules that have a polygonal shape. Certain choroid areas with roughly geometric forms have early filling while other even adjacent areas fill at a very late phase. This is the result of the topography of choroid circulation that is supplied by the short ciliary arteries whose branches are not interlinked (Chapter 1 Fig. 1).

For a certain percentage of cases, the various elements of the choroid are not visible individually but the filling is uniform. Filling of the choriocapillaris is total in five seconds. In some individuals, a dynamic difference can be highlighted in the filling of the districts supplied by the two ciliary arteries. The temporal side of the choroid fills earlier than the nasal hemichoroid. In this way, the watershed between the two territories, that is vertical and passes slightly temporal to the papilla, can be seen.

In the later phases, when the retinal fluorescence has almost disappeared, geographic map structures may again be observed for the residual fluorescence of the choriocapillaris. Indeed, the choriocapillaris normally lets the dye leak through, giving a light diffuse hyperfluorescence while the greater venous vessels of the choroid, that are already empty by that stage, appear to be darker. At the macula, however, it is generally not possible to observe the choroid because of the greater pigmentation of the pigment epithelium and of the presence of the xanthophyllic pigment; for two or three hours after the beginning of the fluorescein angiography a slight choroid and scleral fluorescence persists due to the leaking of fluorescein through the walls of the choroid capillaries.

PART II

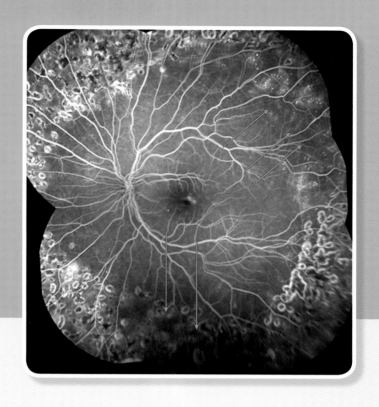

General Principles for Interpreting a Pathological Fluorescein Angiography

Interpreting a Pathological Fluorescein Angiography

The fundamental role of fluorescein angiography is to highlight any alterations of the blood-retinal barrier. Normal retinal capillaries and the greater choroid vessels are watertight to fluorescein while the latter leaks through the walls of the choriocapillaris. This diffusion is, however, masked by the pigment epithelium as its tight junction points that are watertight.

Therefore, there are two blood-retinal barriers: the inner barrier (endothelium of the retinal capillaries) and the outer barrier (retinal pigment epithelium).

Bearing this basic principle in mind, the fluorescein angiography interpretation must be made in two steps:
1. Analytic study
2. Synthetic study.

ANALYTIC STUDY

The analysis of the various elements of a fluorescein angiogram comprises the study of:
- **Abnormal hyperfluorescence:**
    1. Abnormal transmission of fluorescence
    2. Fluorescein leakage or diffusion
    3. Fluorescein pooling
    4. Tissue staining
- **Abnormal hypofluorescence:**
    1. Masking normal fluorescence (screen effect)
    2. Relative or total hypoperfusion of choroid and retinal vessels
- **Abnormalities of retinal and choroid circulation**
    1. Faster transit
    2. Delays in fluorescein clearance
    3. Filling abnormalities
    4. Prolonged hyperfluorescence
- **Localization of changes in the blood-ocular barrier.**

SYNTHETIC EVALUATION

The synthetic evaluation is the most important step in a fluorescein angiographic study because only a synthetic study of the various data analyzed makes it possible to reach a precise and reliable diagnosis. However, the synthetic evaluation also comprises data that are not directly linked to the fluorescein angiography: in order to correctly interpret a fluorescein angiography, it is necessary to know the patient history, have a picture of the fundus with red-free light, know what the visual acuity of the patient is, visual field, blue light photographs, fundus autofluorescence examination, cross section and "en face" OCT, microperimetry. Synthesis needs the help of other examination results.

It is necessary to study all the sequences of the various phases of the fluorescein angiography, the hyperfluorescence and hypofluorescence elements that have been analyzed and the dynamic factors must be compared. If possible, the results of the fluorophotometry. It is *important,* and at times mandatory, to reconstruct the entire retina through photomontage, manual or automatic, and not be content with seeing each frame separately. In this way, it is possible to highlight pathologic aspects of the choroid and of the retina that would otherwise be meaningless when looked at in an isolated frame. Retinal periphery reconstruction is very important in cases of possible peripheral non-perfusion as in diabetic retinopathy and sickle cell retinopathy (Figs 1 and 2).

It is also indispensable to anatomically locate the site of the hypofluorescence or hyperfluorescence. And finally, it is necessary to link abnormal variations of fluorescence with any alterations in the blood-ocular barrier.

It must also be pointed out that in some cases, a normal fluorescein angiography may correspond to an abnormal ocular fundus, and an apparently normal ocular fundus may correspond to an abnormal fluorescein angiography.

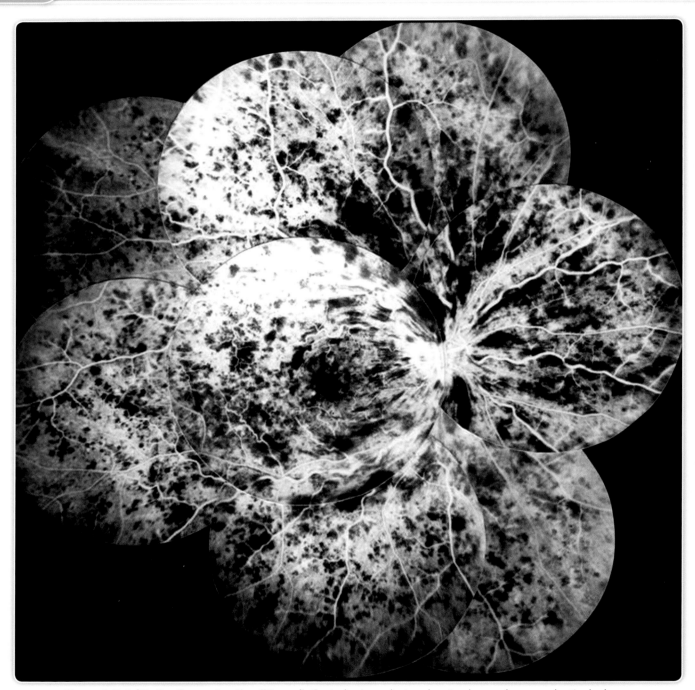

Figure 1: Total Retina Reconstruction (Manual). Central vein occlusion showing hemorrhages and retinal edema.

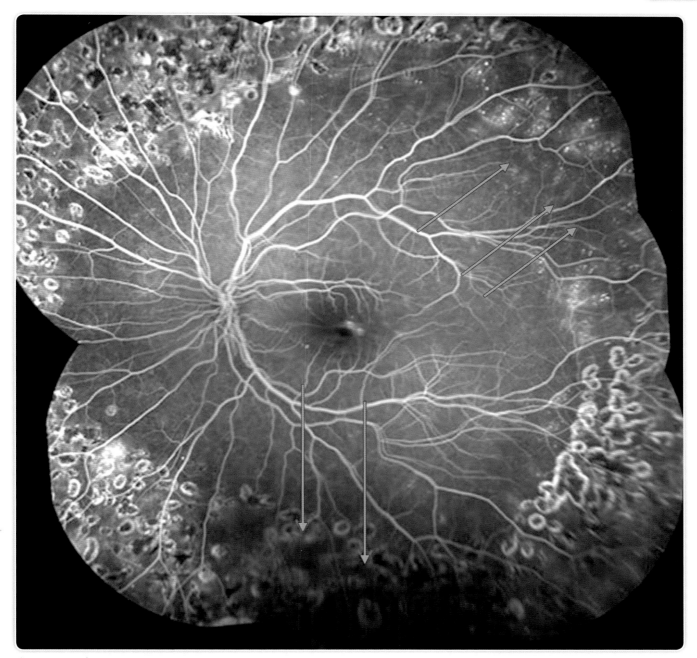

Figure 2: Total Retina Reconstruction (Automatic). Diabetic retinopathy: the central retina shows some microaneurysms, while retinal periphery has been partially treated with laser spots. Some areas have not yet been treated and we can see the ischemic retina (arrows). It is important, and at times mandatory, to make a reconstruction of the entire retina through photomontage, manual or automatic, and not be content with seeing each frame separately. By reconstructing all retina, it is possible to highlight pathologic aspects of the choroid and of the retina that would otherwise be meaningless when looked at in an isolated frame. Retinal periphery reconstruction is very important in cases of possible peripheral non-perfusion as in diabetic retinopathy and sickle cell retinopathy.

PART III

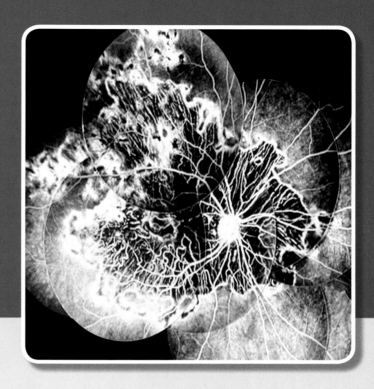

Pathological Fluorescein Angiography Analytical Study

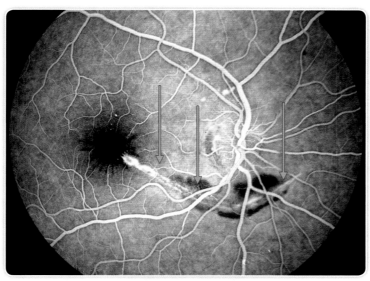

Figure 8A: Anomalous Transmission of Fluorescence. Window Defect. Traumatic Lesions. The rupture of the choroid produces an arcuate window effect with concavity towards the papilla (arrows). In this case, the lesion is inferior to the optic disc. We can still see some hemorrhage at the macula where neovascularization is beginning to develop.

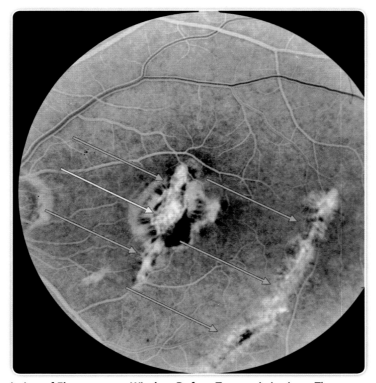

Figure 8B: Anomalous Transmission of Fluorescence. Window Defect. Traumatic Lesions. The rupture of the choroid produces here two arcuate concentric lesions (arrows) with window effect whose concavity is towards the optic disc. In this case, we see hemorrhage at the posterior pol. Neovascularization developed in the macula (yellow arrow).

that diffuses the fluorescein appears at the beginning in the early phases of the fluorescein angiography as a small hyperfluorescent spot whose intensity increases progressively in the following phases as does its size; its edges are never sharply outlined. In the later phases, there generally persists some hyperfluorescence with indefinite boundaries whose intensity progressively decreases.

RETINAL LEAKAGE

Among the retinal leaks mention will be made first of the leakage from ruptures of the external blood-retina barrier and then of the vascular retinal alterations (internal blood-retina barrier).

Central Serous Chorioretinopathy

The origin of the leakage is due to a lesion located at level of the watertight junctions of the retinal pigment epithelium. Generally, the angiography highlights a hyperfluorescent and often isolated spot that appears in the early phases and increases progressively. The typical aspect takes then the shape of an "umbrella", a "fountain", or a "pine-tree" due to the diffusion of the dye in the fluid of the retinal detachment caused by convection currents. At times, instead, the diffusion is more even, centrifugal and has the aspect of a "headlight in the fog". Clinical variations are frequent with multiple leakage points, serous elevation of the pigmented epithelium, etc. (Figs 9 to 13A and B).

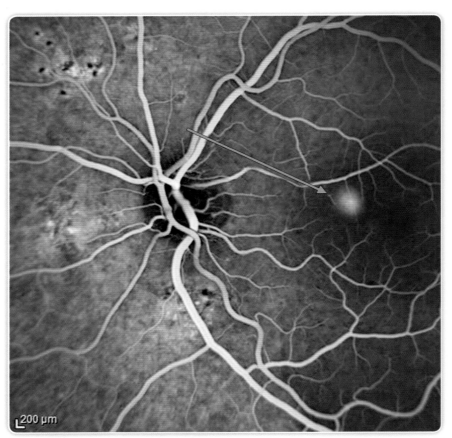

Figure 9: Retinal Leakage in Central Serous Chorioretinopathy. The leakage origins from a lesion located in the watertight junctions of the pigment epithelium. The angiography highlights a hyperfluorescent isolated spot that appears in the early phases and increases progressively. In this case, the diffusion is regular, centrifugal and has the aspect of a "headlight in the fog" (arrow).

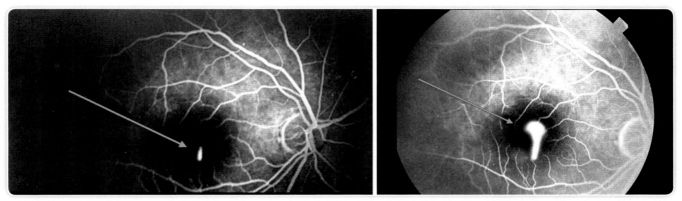

Figure 10: **Retinal Leakage in Central Serous Chorioretinopathy.** The angiography shows a hyperfluorescent isolated spot that appears in the early phases and increases progressively. In a later phase the leakage forms an "umbrella", a "fountain", or a "pine-tree" due to the diffusion of the dye in the fluid of the retinal elevation (arrow).

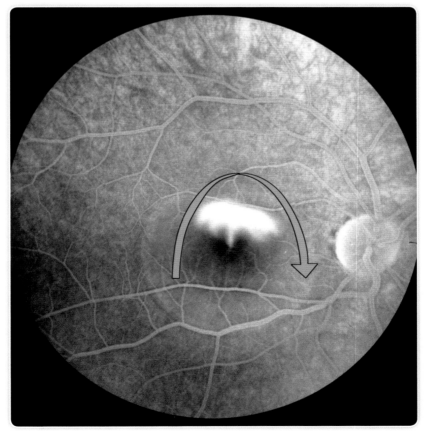

Figure 11: Retinal Leakage in Central Serous Chorioretinopathy. Typical aspect of a "pine-tree" due to the diffusion of the dye in the fluid of the retinal elevation. The dye diffuses from the RPE lesion into the retinal detachment. Due to convection currents, when it reaches the bubble superior limits, it has to follow the detachment borders and flow, first laterally and then down (arrow).

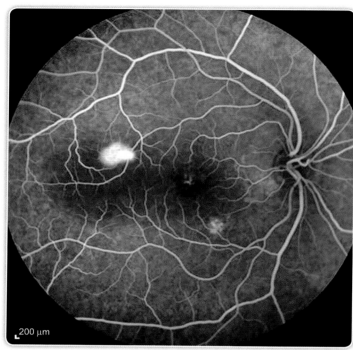

Figure 12: Retinal Leakage in Central Serous Chorioretinopathy. The figure shows a hyperfluorescent isolated spot that appears in the early phases and increases progressively with a regular, centrifugal diffusion and typical aspect of "headlight in the fog".

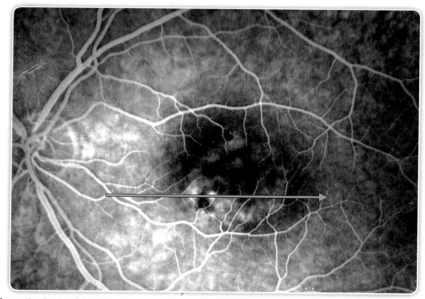

Figure 13A: Retinal Leakage in Central Serous Chorioretinopathy: Fluorescein Angiography. The fluorescein angiography shows an hyperfluorescent spot in the early phases, increasing progressively in the later phases. The arrow shows where the OCT scan has been made.

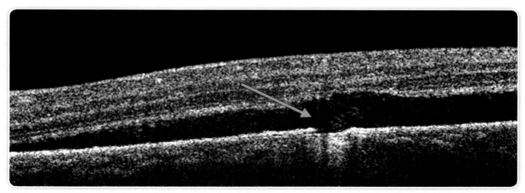

Figure 13B: Retinal Leakage in Central Serous Chorioretinopathy. Cross Section OCT. Same case. The OCT passing exactly through the RPE leaking lesion shows a small fibrin cloud leaking and entering the retinal elevation (arrow).

Chronic Serous Chorioretinopathy

This form is observed in elder patients, and shows larger lesions that combine leakage dots similar to the central serous chorioretinopathy, with less intense leakage points, with scar alterations of the pigment epithelium, and serous detachments of the pigment epithelium. Underlying these two syndromes there is a diffuse, progressive, disorder of the pigment epithelium with acute peaks from time to time.

Harada's Disease

Not frequent in northern Europe, this acute choroiditis shows some multiple retinal serous detachments with intense leakage of the fluorescein. This is often associated with serous elevations of the pigment epithelium and, at times, a large retinal elevation.

Similar leakage cases have been described in patients with exudative choroiditis.

Leakage from Newly Formed Retinal Vessels

Newly formed retinal vessels, whatever their etiology, are characterized by an immature endothelial layer. Leakage from abnormal vascular walls is intense and occurs at an early stage. In the arterial phase, the vessels appear to be sharp and are clearly delineated by the dye, while a small fraction of a second later, the leakage of the fluorescein is intense and completely conceals the morphology of the new vessels (Figs 14 and 15).

Microaneurysms

At a certain point of their evolution, the walls of microaneurysms may allow the fluorescein to leak evenly as a light in the fog.

Venous Occlusion Lesions of the Main Vessels with Leakage

In venous occlusions, obviously after the venous phase, staining of the walls of the major vessels appear and then dye leakage. This leakage increases progressively in the later phases and infiltrates the surrounding retina. As usual, the leakage edges are very blurred.

Leakage in Vasculitis

A localized hyperfluorescence due to staining is noted on the vessel walls with leaks from specific points. The leaks allow the dye to penetrate into the surrounding retina, it increases in the later phases and may persist for over an hour (Fig. 16).

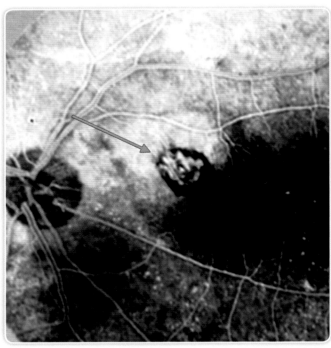

Figure 14: Retinal Leakage CNV Sub-Retinal New Vessels. The fluorescein angiography highlights only a hyperfluorescent small net with intense leakage of the dye (arrow). This aspect is clearly evident in the earlier phases. Deep choroidal hemorrhages may be seen. In the later phases, there will be intense leakage of the dye.

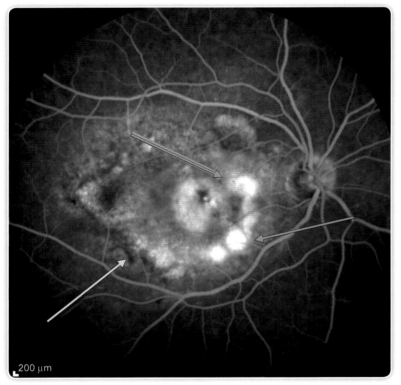

Figure 15: Retinal Leakage CNV Sub-Retinal New Vessels. The figure shows a few highly hyperfluorescent spots with intense leakage of the dye (arrows). Deep choroidal hemorrhages are present as is seen a flat retinal serous detachments (yellow arrow).

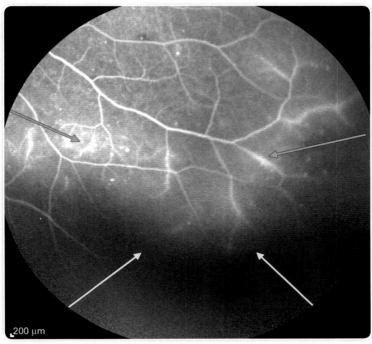

Figure 16: Leakage in Vasculitis. Localized hyperfluorescence due to staining is noted on the vessel walls with leakage from a few specific points (arrows). The leakage allows the dye to penetrate into the surrounding retina, it increases in the later phases and may persist for over an hour. In periphery, non-perfused areas are clearly seen (yellow arrows).

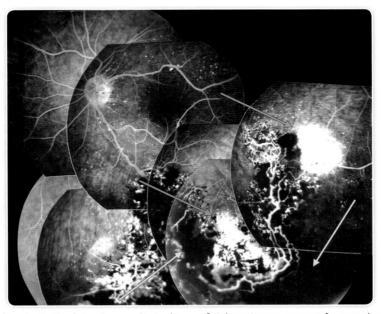

Figure 17: Leakage and Pooling in Retinal Angiomas. Retinal superficial angiomas are not frequently observed in everyday clinical work. They lead, if not treated, to vitreal hemorrhages. In this case, angiomas are located in the inferior temporal retina. Localized hyperfluorescence due to pooling in some places and to leakage (arrows) in other is noted on the angioma lesions walls with leakage from specific points. The leakage increases in the later phases. Some areas are not perfused (yellow arrows). Some capillary walls are intensely stained by the dye.

Leakage and Pooling in Retinal Angiomas

Retinal superficial angiomas are not frequently observed in everyday clinical work, differently from choroidal angiomas that are more frequent. They lead, if not treated, to vitreal hemorrhages. Retinal angioma shows localized hyperfluorescence due to pooling in some places and to leakage in other points. The leakage increases in the later phases. Some areas are not perfused. Capillary walls are intensely stained by the dye (Fig. 17).

CHOROID LEAKAGE

Exudative Choroidopathies

In the acute form, there is an intense subretinal diffusion in relation to the inflammation of the choriocapillaris elements involved.

Sub-retinal New Vessels

The best images of subretinal vessels may be observed when the thinning of the pigmented epithelium enables perfect visualization. In the first phases, the fluorescein angiography highlights only a hyperfluorescent dot with marked leakage of the dye. At this phase a diagnostic error is possible because the lesion looks very much like the leakage spot of a central serous chorioretinopathy. The OCT will solve the problem. A few days later a neovascular network may be observed consisting of a central stalk with branches ending in peripheral anastomoses. The overall aspect is like a bicycle wheel or a fan with fine arborizations. This aspect is clearly evident in the earlier phases. Deep choroidal hemorrhages may often be seen. In the later phases, the vascular network is hidden by the intense leakage of the dye and, at times, by a serous detachment.

Table 6: Causes of vasculitis giving leakage lesions

General infections
Toxoplasmosis
Tuberculosis
Cytomegalovirus
Lyme disease
Herpes simplex
Herpes Zoster- Varicella
Brucellosis
Cat scratch disease
Focal frosted branch angiitis secondary to
    Antistreptolysin O
    Epstein-Barr virus
    Coxsackie virus A10
    Adenovirus
    Measles
    Rubella
    Behçet's disease
Other infections

Systemic diseases
Behçet disease
Sarcoidosis
Lupus erythematosus
Arteritis nodosa
Multiple sclerosis
Leukemia
Crohn's disease,
Other systemic diseases
AIDS retinitis
Systemic lupus erythematosus
Large cell lymphoma and acute lymphoblastic leukemia

Table 7: Causes of serous elevation of the retina

Frequent
- Central serous chorioretinopathy
- Diffuse retinal epitheliopathy
- Macular degenerations
- Subretinal neovascularization
- Optic pits
- Dome shaped macula
- Diabetic retinopathy

Less frequent
- Venous occlusion
- Macular pucker, vitreoretinal traction
- Vitreoretinal interface syndrome
- Epiretinal membranes
- Venous occlusion
- Choroiditis

Rare
- Harada's disease
- Coats' disease
- Angiomatoses
- Choroidal neoformations : Nevi, angioma, melanoma, metastasis
- Sub-retinal parasitosis cysts

Table 8: Differential diagnosis of the central serous chorioretinopathy

- Serous chorioretinopathy
- Incipient subretinal neovascularization
- Serous detachment associated with colobomatous optic pit
- Serous detachment associated with nevi of the choroid
- Dome shaped macula

Table 9: Vascular hyperfluorescence

Retina
- Retinal, preretinal and vitreous neovessels
- Microaneurysms
- Macroaneurysms
- Vascular malformations
- Retinal angiomas
- Wall staining of vasculitis (arteries and veins)
- Arteriovenous anastomoses
- Frost branch angiitis

Choroid
- Subretinal neovascularization
- Choroid angiomas, etc.
- Melanoma
- Metastases

Table 10: Causes of retinal and papillary neovascularization: extensive retinal ischemias

Frequent causes
Diabetic retinopathy
Occlusions of the central retinal vein
Occlusions of the venous branches
Eales' disease
Other forms of vasculitis
Pars planitis
Sickle cell anemia
Thalassemia

Rare causes
Leukemia
Hyperviscosity of crioglobulinemia
Waldenstrom's disease
Multiple myeloma
Very rare or unknown causes

Table 11: Causes of subretinal neovascular membranes

Frequent
Age-related macular degeneration
Idiopathic polypoidal vasculopathy
Retinal angiomatous proliferations (RAP)
Myopia
Idiopathic new vessels in young patients
Pseudohistoplasmosis
Traumatic choroidal ruptures
Complications of laser photocoagulation
Angioid streaks

Rare
Choroiditis
Choroidal nevus
Osteoma
Pseudovitelliform macular dystrophy
Stargardt disease

Table 12: Causes of subretinal neovascularization according to frequency

Age-related macular degeneration
Disciform macular degeneration
Other macular degenerations
Myopia
New vessels in young individuals
Traumatic rupture of Bruch's membrane
Traumatic rupture of choroid
Outcomes of photocoagulation
Angioid streaks
Choroidal nevi

Rare
　　Stargardt
　　Pseudovitelliform degeneration
　　Histoplasmosis
　　Other choroidal inflammation
　　Various causes

Table 13: Intraretinal cavities without leakage in fluorescein angiography

- Vitreomacular traction
- X-linked retinoschisis
- Retinitis pigmentosa
- Telangiectasis cavities
- Nicotinic acid maculopathy
- Juxtafoveal macular telangiectasis
- Outer retinal tubulation
- Fovea vitreomacular traction
- Closed macular hole after surgery
- Achromatopsia
- Alkyl nitrite abuse

FLUORESCEIN POOLING

The pooling of fluorescein in a cystic or pseudo-cystic cavity produces an hyperfluorescence with sharp rounded edges that in time increase in intensity but not in extension; these areas have different sizes: they may be small but they may even be larger than one papilla diameter.

Retinal Pigment Epithelium Serous Detachment

This is a pigment epithelium **detachment** which elevates from Bruch's membrane. The fluid originating from the choriocapillaris pools in the subepithelial space. Fluorescein angiography highlights a fluorescent area

Table 14: Hyperfluorescence III
POOLING
Retina
Idiopathic or secondary elevation of the pigment epithelium
Cystoid edema
Retinal vessels
Microaneurysms
Macroaneurysms
Telangiectasis
Vascular malformations
Coats
Von Hippel Lindau
Choroid
Angiomas
Melanomas
Optic disc
Coloboma
Optic pit

Table 15: Causes of pigment epithelium detachments
Frequent
• Idiopathic elevation single or multiple
• Acute central serous chorioretinopathy
• Chronic diffuse retinal epitheliopathy
• Age-related macular degeneration, with CNV
Rare
• Subretinal new vessels of other origin
Subretinal parasitosis
• Choroidal tumors
Angioid streaks

that appears very early (choroidal phase) and shows sharp rounded edges. Hyperfluorescence within the lesion increases rapidly in the arterial phase, without increasing its surface and persists for hours with marked hyperfluorescence when the other retinal structures have lost their fluorescence. The dye may not be uniformly distributed but be interrupted by "Y" or "H" shaped lines. The serous elevation may be idiopathic, associated with central serous chorioretinopathy, secondary to age-related macular degeneration or serous-hemorrhagic disciform degeneration or secondary to other causes: myopia, angioid streaks, choroiditis, choroid neoformations, etc. (Figs 18 and 19A and B).

Pooling in Retinal Vascular Alterations

Fluorescein may pool in the *microaneurysms*, rounded capillary dilations that dye fills in the early phases and that remain hyperfluorescent well into the later phases. Pooling is possible also in the macroaneurysms of the retinal telangiectasis, in Coat's disease where major elevation of the cavity appear (especially in children) with intense hyperfluorescence. In von Hippel's disease fluorescein angiography highlights a marked early hyperfluorescence of the angiomas. The early phases make it possible to distinguish between the artery and the vein that at times are so dilated that they are not readily recognized (Figs 20 and 21).

Cystoid Macular Edema

In cystoid macular edema we see chronic pooling of intraretinal fluid in pseudocystic formations or intraretinal cavities arranged around the fovea. Its aspect has been likened to the petals of a flower or honeycomb. Initially, the fovea is not involved. However, later, a central loggia may appear that entails a marked and final decrease in the vision. Fluorescein angiography, the cavities of the cystoid macular edema form a screen against the normal fluorescence in the earlier phases, and then pooling spots appear issuing from the posterior pole capillaries. In the later phases, the aspect is typical with the hyperfluorescent pseudocystic cavities flower shaped around the foveal area. Cystoid edema remains highly hyperfluorescent even in the later phases up to one or two hours from the beginning of the fluorescein examination. At this point, the pseudocysts have blurred edges with slight dye leakage. The causes of cystoid macular edema are listed in a separate table (Figs 22 and 23A to C).

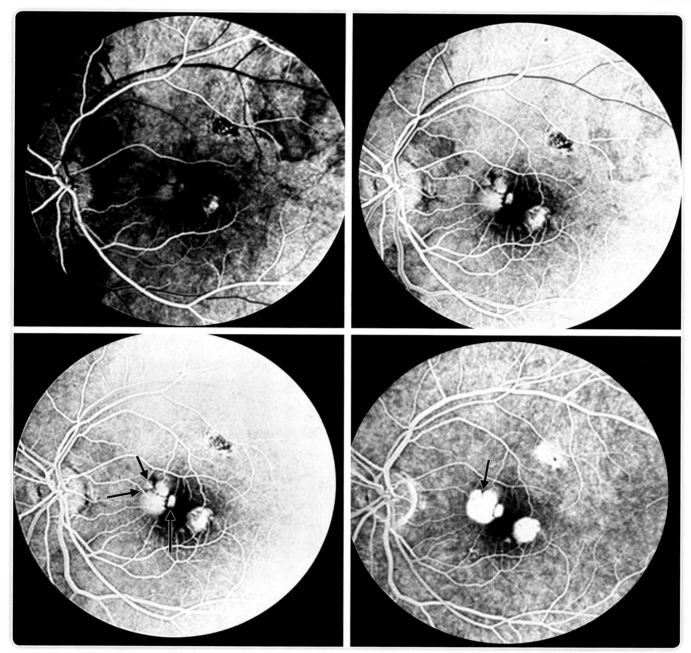

Figure 18: Pooling Pigment Epithelium Detachment (PED). The figure shows four **detachments** of the pigment epithelium, which detachs itself from Bruch's membrane. The fluid from the choriocapillaris pools in the subepithelial space.

Fluorescein angiography highlights a fluorescent area that appears very early (choroidal phase) with sharp roundish edges. Hyperfluorescence within the lesion increases rapidly in the arterial phase, without leakage and persists for hours with marked hyperfluorescence while the other retinal structures have lost their fluorescence. The dye is not uniformly distributed but be interrupted by "Y" or "H" shaped pigment lines (arrow). The serous detachment in this case is idiopathic. It could be associated chronic central serous chorioretinopathy, secondary to serous-hemorrhagic disciform degeneration or secondary to rarer causes: myopia, angioid streaks, choroiditis, choroid neoformations, etc.

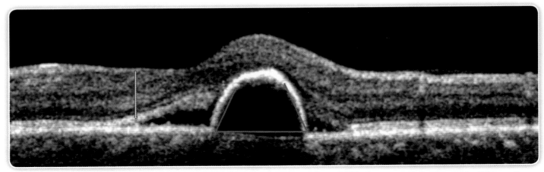

Figure 19A: Pooling; Pigment Epithelium Detachment (PED). Cross section OCT shows a detachment of the pigment epithelium that elevates itself from Bruch's membrane with an angle of more than 45° (arrows). The fluid from the choriocapillaris pools in the subepithelial space. Here we see also a small detachment of the neuro retina (yellow arrow).

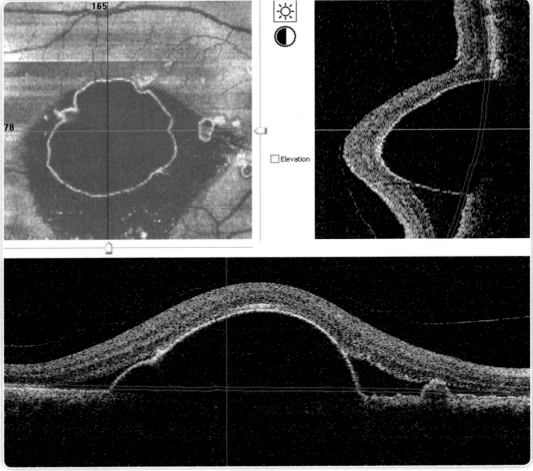

Figure 19B: Pooling; Pigment Epithelium Detachment (PED). "En face" OCT shows a detachment of the pigment epithelium . The walls are thin and smooth, the shape is circular.

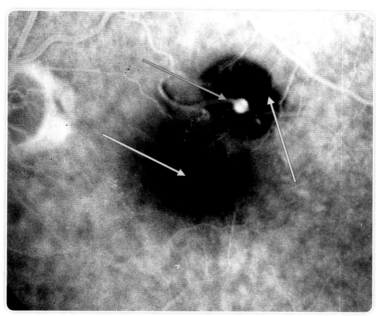

Figure 20: Pooling in Retinal Vascular Alterations Macroaneurysms. Macroaneurysms are much bigger than microaneurysms. Pooling is possible in the macroaneurysms and their cavity appear intensely hyperfluorescent (arrow). Dense dark hemorrhages surround the vascular lesion (yellow arrow). They are frequently seen in senior patients affected with hypertension or atherosclerosis.

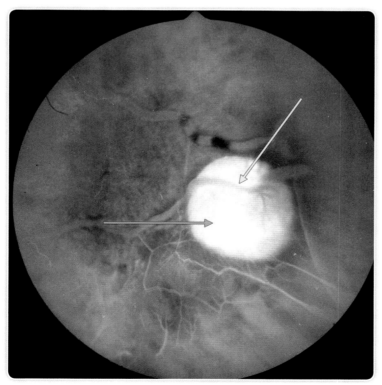

Figure 21: Pooling in Retinal Vascular Alterations. Von Hippel's disease. In von Hippel's disease fluorescein angiography highlights an intense early hyperfluorescence of the angioma (arrow). During the early phases, it is possible to distinguish between the afferent artery (yellow arrow) and the vein that at times are so dilated that they are not readily recognized.

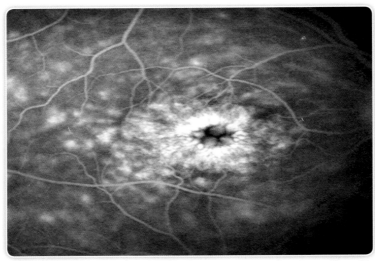

Figure 22: Pooling. Cystoid Macular Edema. In cystoid macular edema, we can see chronic pooling of intraretinal fluid in pseudocystic formations or intraretinal cavities arranged around the fovea. Its aspect has been likened to the petals of a flower. A centralcavity may appear that entails a marked and final decrease in the visual acuity. Fluorescein angiographically, the cysts of the cystoid macular edema form a screen against the normal fluorescence in the earlier phases, and then the dye pools inside the cavities in the late phases. Later leakage appears starting from the capillaries of the posterior pole. In the later phases the aspect is typical with the hyperfluorescent pseudocysts flower shaped around the foveal area. The biggest cavities are localized at the fovea. Cystoid edema remains very hyperfluorescent even in the later phases up to one or two hours from the beginning of the test. At this point the pseudocysts show blurred edges with leakage of the dye.

Table 16: Fluorescein pooling
• Retinal pigment epithelium serous detachment
• Microaneurysms
• Macroaneurysms
• Cystoid edema
• Von Hippel

Table 17: Hyperfluorescence IV
Staining
Retina
Diffused or localized edema
Retinal vessel walls
Vasculitis
Venous occlusions
Abnormal vessels
Arteriovenous shunts
Neoformations
Angiomas
Malformations
Pigment epithelium and Bruch's membrane
Placoid epitheliopathy
Serpiginous epitheliopathy
Drusen
Chorioretinal scars
Choroid
Neoformations

Pooling in the Choroid

In some choroid tumors, there may be pooling especially in angiomas of the choroid where the fundus indistinct neoformation stains rapidly and its hyperfluorescence persists until the later phases.

In some melanomas of the choroid, we can see hyper-fluorescent areas due to the pooling of dye (Figs 24A and B).

In case of optic pit of the papilla a marked hyperfluorescence can be noted due to pooling of the fluorescence.

TISSUE STAINING

Fluorescein staining of the tissues is seen in fluorescein angiography as a hyperfluorescence that begins in the early venous phase, the edges are blurred and its intensity and extension increase little in the later angiographic phases.

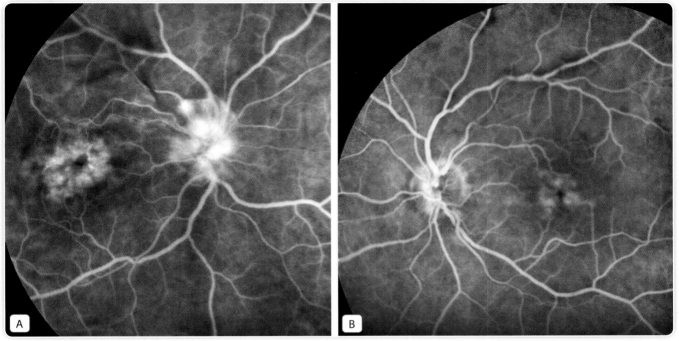

Figures 23A and B: Pooling. Cystoid Macular Edema in Cases of Postoperative Cystoid Edema (Irvine Gass Syndrome). The pseudocysts show blurred edges. Optic disc hyperfluorescence is clearly seen.

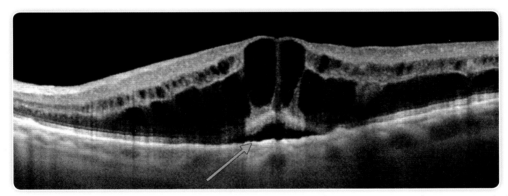

Figure 23C: Pooling. Cystoid Macular Edema—Cross Section OCT. Edema pseudocysts are seen in the inner macular layer, where they are small, and in the outer macular layer, where they are bigger. A small retinal serous detachment is localized at the fovea(arrow). The serous retina detachments cannot be seen on fluorescein angiographs.

Retina

In diffuse or localized retinal edema, the fluorescein spreads from the vascular walls, staining the retinal tissue without any pooling of the dye. The starting point may be a diffused vascular alteration, as occurs in acute arterial hypertension in young people, or diabetic microangiopathy (Fig. 25).

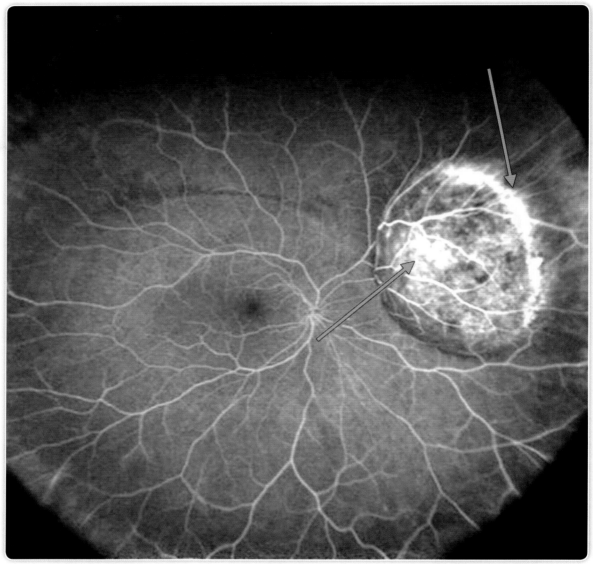

Figure 24A: Pooling. Choroidal Melanoma. Fluorescein Angiography. Pooling in a case of choroidal melanoma. Underneath normal retinal vessels, an abnormal dye accumulation can be seen in the tumor mass. In this case, however, while in the early phases of the fluorescein angiography the screen is total, in the later stages the neoformation is irregularly fluorescent (arrows).

Staining of the Vascular Walls

In some cases of venous occlusion, in retinal arteritis and phlebitis, marked arterial or venous staining may be noticed. Some vessel segments may be highly hyperfluorescent with slightly blurred edges. The staining may extend to the surrounding retina. Hyperfluorescence may persist up to one or two hours after the beginning of the angiogram. In some vascular malformations (angiomas), the surrounding edematous tissues may stain. The abnormal vessels of the arterio-venous anastomoses that are observed after certain retinal occlusions show intensely stained walls (Fig. 26).

The retinal drusen, that at the early phases of the fluorescein angiography present a window effect hyperfluorescence, will later stain with dye and preserve the fluorescence into the later phases.

• Some chorioretinal scars present staining.

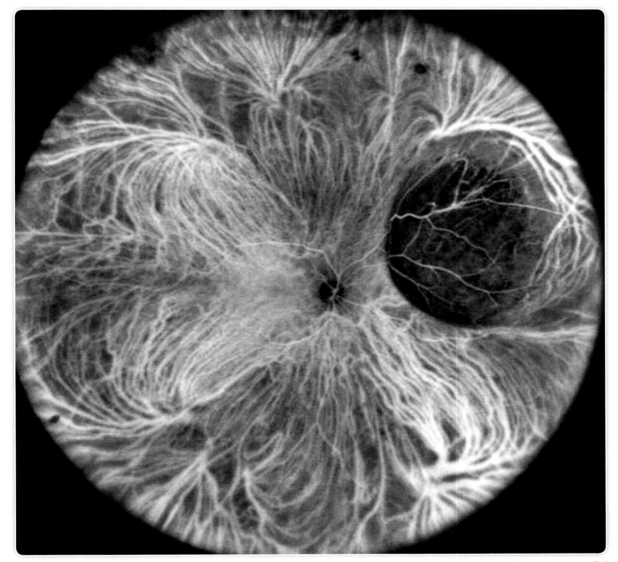

Figure 24B: Pooling. Choroidal Melanoma. Indocyanine Green Angiography with Wide Angle Lens. Pooling in a case of choroidal melanoma. Under normal retinal vessels, abnormal dye accumulation can be seen in the mass of the tumor.

Table 18: Causes of retinal microaneurysms
Diabetic retinopathy
Venous occlusions
Sickle cell disease
Hypertensive retinopathy
Peripheral telangiectasis
Coat's disease
Eales' disease
Vitreoretinal interface disorders
Some microaneurysms can be seen in retinal periphery in apparently normal persons

Table 19: Causes of macroaneurysms
Arterial sclerosis
Hypertensive retinopathy

Table 20: Differential diagnosis of microaneurysms
Microaneurysm: Immediate staining, round with sharp edges, complete filling, slight leakage, surrounding retinal edema
Drusen: Slower staining with slight increase in fluorescence in the later phases; staining, no leakage and no retinal edema

Table 21: Differential diagnosis of a small RPE elevation

Small serous elevation of retina

Polypoidal choroidopathy

Drusen

Limited disruption of the IS/OS junction (ellipsoid)

Table 22: Causes of cystoid macular edema

Frequent causes
Diabetic retinopathy
Venous occlusions (central vein or branch occlusion)
Age-related macular degeneration
Irvine Gass's postsurgery syndrome
Pars planitis
Uveitis
Iridocyclitis
Choroiditis
Bird shot retinopathy
Less frequent causes
Chronic diffuse retinal epitheliopathy
Traction by epiretinal membrane
Retraction of the internal limiting membrane
Vitreoretinal interface syndrome
Macular pucker
Retinitis pigmentosa
Rare
Macular telangiectasis
Coat's disease
Leber's disease
Macroaneurysms
Retinal and choroidal neoformations
Retinal angioma
Hamartoma
Choroidal angioma
Melanoma
Metastatic tumors
Osteoma
Choroidal nevus
   Epinephrine drops
   Radiation retinopathy
   Retinal surgery
Other causes

Table 23: Causes of regressive cystoid edema

Long standing diabetic retinopathy
Long standing macular degeneration non-treated
Long standing venous occlusion non-treated
Diabetic retinopathy treated by laser for more than 5 years
Diabetic retinopathy repeatedly treated by anti-VEGF
Venous occlusion repeatedly treated by anti-VEGF
Age-related macular degeneration repeatedly treated by anti-VEGF
Macular telangiectasis

Table 24: Causes of retinoschisis

Juvenile sex linked macular retinoschisis
Peripheral retinoschisis of the adult
Retinoschisis in high myopia
Goldmann Favre vitreo tapetoretinal degeneration
Retinoschisis secondary to
   Traction
   Impending hole
   Optic pit
Wagner vitreoretinopathy

Table 25: Causes of localized or diffuse macular edemas

Diabetic retinopathy
Venous occlusions (R.C.V. Or branches)
Artery occlusions
Hypertensive retinopathy
Gravidic toxemia
Uveitis
Iridocyclitis
Vitreoretinal interface syndrome
Retraction of the internal limiting membrane
Traction by epiretinal membrane
Retinitis pigmentosa
Optic pit

Table 26: Differential diagnosis of cystoid macular edema

Microcystic degeneration
X-linked retinoschisis
Myopic retinoschisis
Traumatic (surgical) retinoschisis
Non-exudative edemas
Macular pseudo-holes
Hole in formation
Retinal serous elevation
Telangiectasis cavities

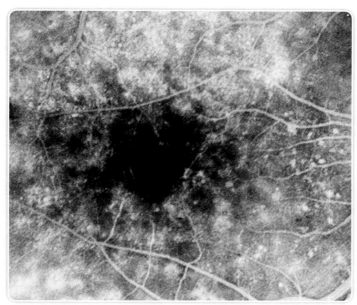

Figure 25: Staining. Retina Staining. Diabetic Microangiopathy. Dye infiltrating ocular tissues results in staining. In diffuse or localized retinal edema, fluorescein spreads from the vascular walls, staining the retinal tissue without any pooling of the dye. The starting point may be a diffuse vascular alteration.

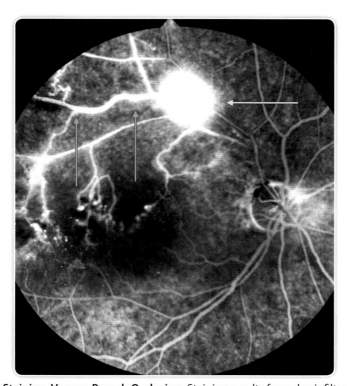

Figure 26: Staining. Vessel Wall Staining. Venous Branch Occlusion. Staining results from dye infiltrating ocular tissues. In this case of venous branch occlusion, a marked arterial or venous staining may be noticed. Some vessel segments are highly hyperfluorescent with slightly blurred edges. The staining in some places extends to the surrounding retina. Hyperfluorescence may persist up to one or two hours from the beginning of the angiogram. The anomalous arterivenous shunts have intensely stained walls (arrows). Note one spot of intense leakage (yellow arrow) due to new formed vessels and the venous occlusion non- perfused areas.

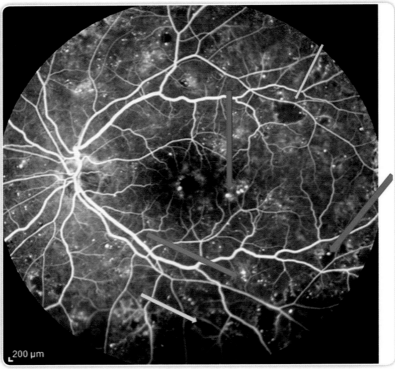

Figure 27: Pooling; Microaneurysms. Fluorescein may pool in the *microaneurysms*, rounded capillary dilations that dye fills in the early phases and that remain hyperfluorescent well into the later phases. Fluorescein angiography can highlight their onset in relationship with arteriolar micro occlusions. Microaneurysms have an evolution that can be seen in this image of diabetic retinopathy. They begin as small vasodilatations, they increase in size, disappear in a given point and then reappear in other places. Incipient microaneurysms are small (arrows) but they can clearly be seen through fluorescein angiography; some are bigger and *fluorescein may leaks* out through their walls (red arrow). Some microaneurysm clusters leaking dye may be seen. Alterations of the macular capillary network are seen as well as some non-perfused small areas (yellow arrows).

Abnormal Hypofluorescence

Table 1: Hypofluorescence

- SCREEN AGAINST NORMAL FLUORESCENCE
- FILLING DEFECT

SCREEN OR MASK EFFECT OF NORMAL FLUORESCENCE

Normal fluorescence of the ocular fundus may be masked at different levels:
- Preretinal (lens opacities and vitreous opacities or vitreous hemorrhage)
- Retina (hemorrhages at different levels of the retina, pigment, foreign bodies, etc.)
- Choroid (hemorrhages, neoformations, etc.)
  The screening elements may be isolated or clustered.

TOTAL SCREEN

Hemorrhages

The most frequent total screen consists of hemorrhages that may be retinal (at various levels of the retina), choroidal or pre-retinal. Preretinal and vitreous hemorrhages hide the fluorescence of the retina and of the choroid. Depending on where they occur, retinal hemorrhages may hide retinal vessels and capillaries. Choroidal hemorrhages instead allow the overlying retinal vessels to be perfectly viewed; there may also be hemorrhagic elevation of the pigmented epithelium.

The choroidal hemorrhages themselves may be more or less deep (Figs 3 to 5).

Pigment

Pigmented formations may form a screen against the normal fluorescence of the choroid.

Table 2: Hypofluorescence I

SCREEN AGAINST NORMAL FLUORESCENCE

Absolute screen	Preretinal, retinal and subretinal hemorrhages Pigment Foreign bodies Pigmented neoformations
Incomplete screen	Opacities of the crystalline lens Hemorrhage of the vitreous Some retinal hemorrhage Exudates
Transient screen	Retinal edema Choroiditis Placoid epitheliopathy Serpiginous epitheliopathy Serous retinal elevation Lipofuscin deposits in Best's disease

Pre-retinal = lens and vitreous opacities

retinal = hemorrhages, pigment

choroid = hemorrhages, pigment, tumors

Table 3: Causes of preretinal hemorrhages

Frequent
Hypertensive retinopathy
Diabetic retinopathy
Venous occlusions
Posterior vitreous detachment
Direct or indirect ocular trauma

Less frequent
Blood dyscrasias
Anemia,
Leukemia
Bacterial endocarditis
Subdural hemorrhage
Subarachnoid hemorrhage
Terson syndrome

Unknown causes

Table 4: Causes of superficial hemorrhages
Posterior pole
Hypertensive retinopathy
Diabetic retinopathy
Venous occlusions
AMD macular degeneration
Unknown causes in young women
Oral contraceptives
Unknown causes
Blood diseases
Dyscrasias
Anemia
Leukemia
Around optic disc
Glaucoma and normal tension glaucoma
Papilledema
Papillitis
Ischemic optic neuropathy
Papillophlebitis

Table 5: Causes of deep hemorrhages
Hypertensive retinopathy
Diabetic retinopathy
Venous occlusions
Lacquer cracks in myopia
AMD macular degeneration
Angioid streaks
Anemia
Leukemia
Blood dyscrasias
Oral contraceptives
Unknown causes

Hyperplasia and hypertrophies of the pigment epithelium are very dense as are certain nevi and melanomas. In this latter case, however, while in the early phases of the fluorescein angiography the screen is total, in the later stages the neoformation is irregularly fluorescent (Figs 1 and 2).

Foreign bodies also constitute a total screen.

INCOMPLETE SCREEN

Constant Screen

Incomplete screens may be constant or transient. Among constant screens there are the lens opacities and the vitreous opacities. Long-standing retinal detachments containing very dense fluid, may constitute a complete or incomplete screen depending on the state of the subretinal fluid.

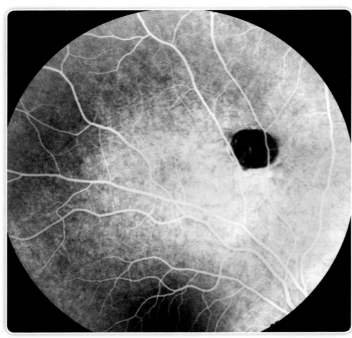

Figure 1: Screen Effect. Pigment Hyperplasia. Hyperplasia of the pigment epithelium may be very dense. Pigmented formations form a screen against the normal fluorescence of the choroid, but the retinal vessels are clearly seen, passing on the black backdrop.

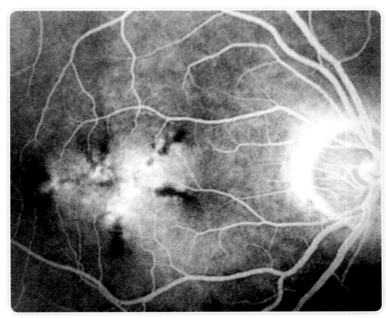

Figure 2: Screen Effect. Pattern Macular Degeneration. Pigment deposits in the retina may form a screen against the normal fluorescence of the choroid. In this case, we see a form of age-related atypical degeneration, the macular pattern degeneration with typically branching pigmented lines. In the fluorescein angiography, the screen is total, in the autofluorescence images the same formation is typically irregularly fluorescent.

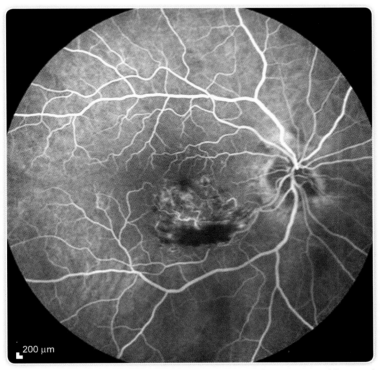

Figure 3: Screen Effect. Superficial Hemorrhage in Branch Venous Occlusion. This pre-retinal hemorrhage hides the fluorescence of the underlying retina and choroid.

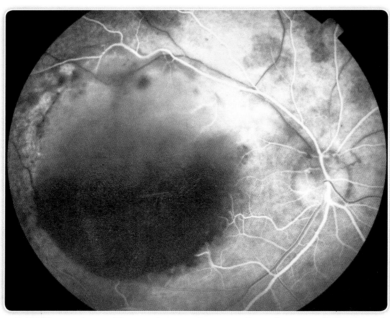

Figure 4: Screen Effect. Superficial Hemorrhage. The total screen here consists of a pre-retinal hemorrhage. Hemorrhage blocks the fluorescence of retinal vessels and capillaries.

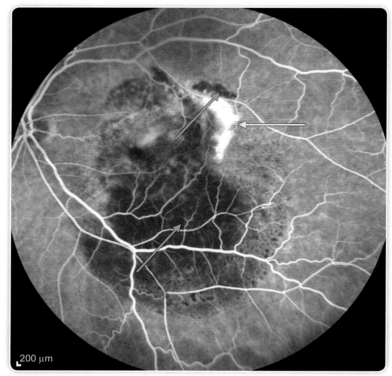

Figure 5. Screen Effect. Deep Hemorrhage. In this AMD case, the choroidal hemorrhages allow the overlying retinal vessels to be perfectly viewed. The choroidal hemorrhages themselves are more or less deep (arrows). The neovascularization may be seen on the border of the hemorrhages as an hyperfluorescent leakage area (yellow arrow).

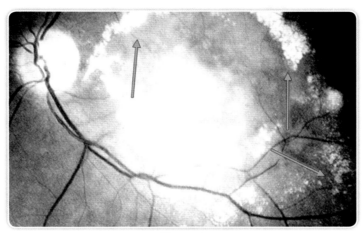

Figure 6

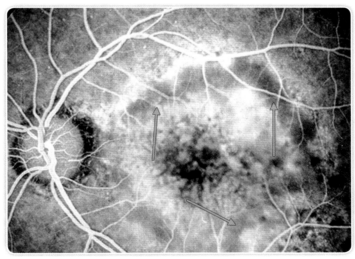

Figure 7

Figures 6 and 7: Screen Effect. Transitory Screen. Hard exudates form a screen in the early phases of the fluorescein angiography, but then in the later phases the screen decreases and becomes incomplete (arrows). Exudates here surround an area of intraretinal microvascular lesions that leak diffuse edema.

TRANSITORY SCREEN

Hard exudates form a screen in the early phases of the fluorescein angiography, but then the screen decreases and becomes incomplete (Figs 6 and 7).

Retinal edema, both simple and cystoid, forms a screen in the earlier phases.

The choroiditis granuloma, in the earlier phases, is sharply hypofluorescent whereas in the later phases it becomes hyperfluorescent with a progressive and persistent staining up to one to two hours from the beginning of the fluorescein angiography.

Table 6: Filling defects
Hyperplasia
Hypertrophy of the pigment epithelium
Nevus
Melanoma
• Diabetic retinopathy
• Hypertensive retinopathy
• Coats' disease
• Macular degeneration
Venous occlusions
• Macular telangiectasis
• Radiation retinopathy

Table 7: Causes of cotton wool exudates

Frequent
Hypertensive retinopathy
Arterial branch occlusion
Radiation retinopathy
Purtscher syndrome
Diabetic retinopathy
Venous occlusions

Rare
Hodgkin
Anemia
Lupus erythematosus
Leptospirosis
Kala-azar

Table 8: Causes of subretinal deposits

Macular degeneration (pigment or lipofuscin)

Lipofuscin deposits in pseudovitelliform maculopathy

Tamoxiphen deposits

Macular atrophy (pigment or disrupted drusen material)

Among the rare screens mention can be made of the lipofuscin deposits seen in Best's disease.

VASCULAR FILLING DEFECTS

Vascular filling defects may be observed both in the retina and in the choroid.

FILLING DEFECTS: RETINA

Artery Occlusion

Fluorescein angiography rarely highlights the occlusions of the central retinal artery.

More frequently branch artery occlusions are seen that, at times, also show the embolus or the atheroma plaque that is responsible for the obstacle to the blood flow, and in the earlier arteriovenous phases, lack of filling of the vascular district involved.

Filling, however, may occur at the later phases, very slowly or through the retrograde pathway.

Capillaritis is a frequent cause of branch artery occlusion (Fig. 8).

Table 9: Hypofluorescence II

Vascular filling defects
- **Retina**
  - A. Occlusion of retinal arteries
  - B. Venous occlusions (ischemic forms)
  - C. Capillary micro-occlusions
    - Diabetic
    - Vasculitis
    - Blood diseases
    - Eales' disease
    - Coat's disease
    - Vascular malformations
- **Choroid**
  Triangular syndromes in the periphery
  Rounded or irregular syndromes in the center
  - A. Inflammation
    - Choroiditis
    - Vasculitis
  - B. Vascular causes
    - Emboli
    - Occlusions
  - C. Trauma
- **Various** (retinal and choroidal)
  - Degenerations
  - Dystrophies
  - Congenital abnormalities
- **Filling abnormalities:** Mention is made here only of retrograde filling of the retinal vessels in the case of artery occlusion and abnormal filling of chorioretinal anastomoses
- **Prolonged fuorescence:** Prolonged fluorescence is observed in all cases of pooling and tissue staining, for instance, in cystoid macular edema or hperfluorescence of the papilla in cases of optical atrophy

Venous Occlusion

In venous occlusions, the fluorescein angiography reveals a marked slowdown in the filling of the venous vessels of the district involved.

In the ischemic forms of central vein occlusion and of branch occlusion vast districts of ischemia can be viewed with dilated shunt vessels with hyperfluorescent wall.

These areas of ischemia may however, in the early weeks, be masked by superficial retinal hemorrhages (Fig. 9).

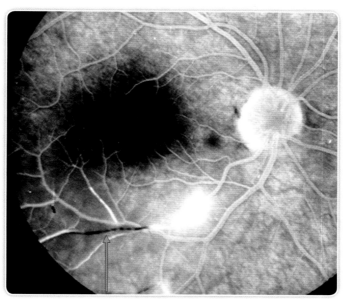

Figure 8: Filling Defects. Branch Artery Occlusion in Capillaritis. In this case of **branch artery occlusion in capillaritis,** we see lack of filling of an artery segment and of the vascular district involved (arrow). Filling, however, occurs at the later phases, very slowly or through the retrograde pathway. A section of the vessel shows intense leakage in vasculitis. Hyperfluorescence due to staining is noted on the vessel walls with leakage from specific segments. Leakage allows the dye to penetrate into the surrounding retina, it increases in the later phases and may persist for over an hour.

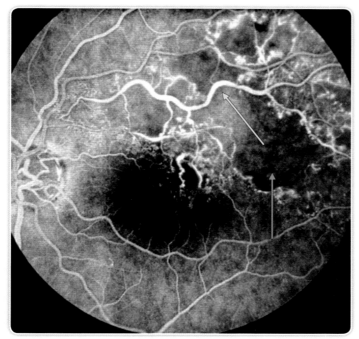

Figure 9: Filling Defects. Branch Vein Ischemic Occlusion. In the venous occlusion area, the capillaries are clearly dilated and tortuous and show intense wall staining (yellow arrow). Some hemorrhages and exudates cover the districts involved. The macular capillary network is affected and visual loss occurs at an early stage. In these forms of venous ischemic branch occlusions, new formed vessels may appear on the edges of the area involved. Localized photocoagulation treatment is required in the areas of non-perfusion (arrow) to avoid hemorrhages and vascular glaucoma.

Capillary Micro-occlusions

Capillary micro-occlusions form one of the most interesting chapters of fluorescein angiography. There are multiple causes for them but the most frequent is **diabetic retinopathy.**

These alterations can be seen also in venous thrombosis, vasculitis, Eale's disease, thalassemia, sickle cell anemia and in other blood disorders (Figs 10 to 12).

The ischemic area is slightly less fluorescent than the normal retina and is more easily noted through contrast between gray normal retina and darker ischemic retina; along its borders there are often seen microaneurysms clusters and frequently dilated capillaries that form arteriovenous shunts or anastomoses.

Hypofluorescence is seen in the capillary phase and is generally maintained in the subsequent phases. In other cases, however, the diffusion of the dye starting from the microaneurysms and from the vascular walls of the surrounding capillaries conceals the hypofluorescence.

Vascular Malformations

In Coat's disease, vascular malformations are often associated with vast areas of hypoperfusion where the residual dilated capillaries have an abnormal course and are particularly evident.

Other Causes

Vascular filling defects may be seen in retinal degeneration, dystrophies, congenital abnormalities (myopia, choroideremia, areolar atrophy of the choroid, etc.) and, also, diathermy or photocoagulation treatment of the retina, Dynamic phototherapy.

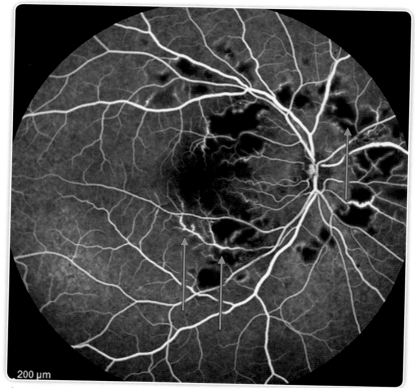

200 μm

Figure 10: Filling Defects. Ischemic Areas and Capillary Micro-occlusions Around the Optic Disc in a Case of Blood Disorder (Moschowitz Disease) in a Young Woman. In this young 20 years old woman, numerous capillary micro-occlusions are seen around the optic disc. The capillary net is less dense than normal. Many capillaries crossing ischemic areas show staining and leakage as in vasculitis (arrows).

FILLING DEFECTS: CHOROID

Vascular filling defects may be seen in choroid after choroid arteries occlusions, mainly the short posterior ciliary arteries. They may be due to:

- Vascular causes: blood diseases, hypertension, emboli, occlusions
- Inflammation: choroiditis, vasculitis
- Blunt traumatisms.

Rarely to degeneration, dystrophies, congenital abnormalities (choroideremia, areolar atrophy of the choroid, etc.) and, also, diathermy or laser treatment of the retina, or dynamic phototherapy.

These defects are polygonal at the posterior pole, triangular in periphery and mid periphery

Table 10: Causes of retinal ischemia
Frequent causes:
• Diabetic retinopathy
• Occlusions of the central retinal vein
• Occlusions of the venous branches
• Eales' disease
• Other vasculitis
• Pars planitis
• Sickle-cell anemia
• Thalassemia
Rare causes:
• Leukemia
• Cryoglobulinemia
• Waldenstrom disease
• Multiple myeloma
• Unknown causes

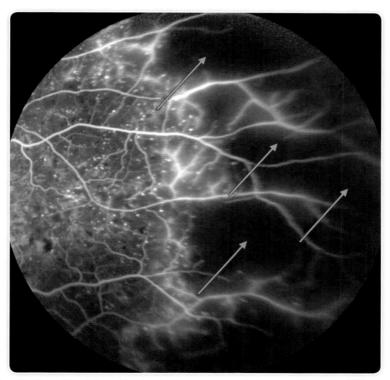

Figure 11: Filling Defects. Non-Perfused Peripheral Retina in Drepanocytosis. We see absence of filling in a large non- perfused zone at periphery (arrows) of the eye. The capillary net is less dense than normal. A part of the capillaries show some staining and leakage as in vasculitis. Hyperfluorescence due to staining is noted on the vessel walls with leakage from specific segments. The leakage allows the dye to penetrate into the surrounding retina. Some microaneurysm clusters are seen close to the non-perfused area.

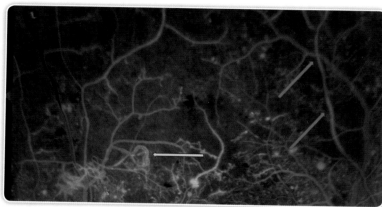

Figure 12: Filling Defects. Diabetic Retinopathy Non-Perfused Areas. Capillary micro-occlusions have multiple causes. In this case, they are observed in a case of diabetic retinopathy. The ischemic districts are slightly less fluorescent than the normal retina and are more evident due to contrast; along non-perfused areas borders dilated capillaries form arteriovenous anastomoses. Numerous microaneurysms cluster close to the non-perfused areas. Some leakage, a few venous dilatations (arrows) and loops (yellow arrow) are observed. Laminar flow in a venous segment indicates a slower blood flow.

Abnormalities in Circulation Time

Abnormalities of circulatory time may be subdivided into: accelerated filling of the vessels, delayed filling, filling abnormalities, prolonged hyperfluorescence.

Table 1: Dynamic abnormalities

Vascular filling defects

I. **Faster filling**
   – Retinal congenital artero-venous anastomoses
   – Arteriovenous anastomoses secondary to branch venous occlusions
   – Retinal angiomas
   – Chorio-retinal anastomoses
   – Choroid hemangiomas
   – Choroid melanomas

II. **Delayed filling**
   A. **Global delay**
      Heart disorders
      Pulmonary congestion
      Carotid stenosis
   B. **Retina**
      Venous occlusions of the CRV or of its branches
   C. **Choroid**
      Physiological irregular filling
      Occlusion of the posterior ciliary vessels
   D. **Optic nerve**
      Ischemic optical disease
      Coloboma
      Optic pit

III. **Retrograde filling**
   Some arterial occlusions
   Chorioretinal anastomoses

IV. **Prolonged fluorescence**
   Pooling
   Cystoid macular edema,
   Microaneurysms
   Macroaneurysms
   Von Hippel syndrome
   Staining
   Localized edema
   Diffuse edema

FASTER VASCULAR FILLING

Faster filling can be noticed in the case of congenital arteriovenous anastomosis. Being connected, arteries and veins skip the capillary phase. Artery-venous anastomoses, secondary to partial venous occlusions both allow for a filling acceleration even though this is in part offset by slower circulation due to the thrombosis.

In retinal angiomas, venous filling is very fast and occurs simultaneously with the capillary filling in the other retinal districts.

Chorioretinal anastomoses show a great rapidity in retinal perfusion.

Choroid hemangiomas are characterized by important vessels that fill rapidly and irregularly with fluorescein during the choroid phase, before arterial filling. Hyperfluorescence is intense, irregular and early.

In some cases of melanoma of the choroid, if there are no major masking phenomena, there is an intense hyperfluorescence due to pooling as early as the choroidal filling.

DELAYED FILLING

There is a delay in the normal filling of the choroid and retina in the presence of major general circulatory disorders such as myocardial diseases, pulmonary congestion, altered viscosity of the blood. In the case of carotid stenosis, perfusion of the choroid and retina on the affected side occurs in 8–10 seconds later than on the non-affected side; and for the late venous phase the difference is more than 20 seconds.

Table 2: Accelerated filling

Congenital arteriovenous anastomosis

Arteriovenous anastomoses, secondary to partial venous occlusions may allow for a filling acceleration

Retinal angiomas

Chorioretinal anastomoses

Choroid hemangiomas

Some cases of melanoma of the choroid

Table 3: Delayed filling

a. **General circulatory disorders** such as
   Myocardial diseases
   Pulmonary congestion
   Altered viscosity of the blood
   Some blood disorders
   Carotid stenosis.

b. **Retina**
   Venous occlusions central vein or branch occlusions.

c. **Choroid**
   Physiological filling delay of the *choriocapillaris* with a mosaic aspect
   Obstruction of the *posterior ciliary vessels.*

d. **Optic nerve**
   Vascular optic disc hypoperfusion with late peripapillary hyperfluorescencee.
   Coloboma of the optic nerve.

Retina

There is a marked slowdown in retinal circulation especially in the venous phases in case of occlusions of the trunk or of the branches of the central retinal vein.

Choroid

There is often a physiological filling delay of the *choriocapillaris* with a mosaic aspect caused by alternation of injected and non-injected zones of the choriocapillaris. In case of obstruction of the *posterior ciliary vessels,* there is delayed filling of the occluded zone. In later stages, because of the anastomoses and retrograde filling, the choroid presents normal fluorescence.

Optic Nerve

In ischemic optic disc disorders, there is early hypofluorescence due to hypoperfusion of the optic disc with late peripapillary hyperfluorescence.

Coloboma will present an early hypofluorescence followed by hyperfluorescence.

FLUORESCEIN ANGIOGRAPHY AND BLOOD-RETINA BARRIER

Table 4: Blood-retinal barrier
- Inner barrier: endothelium of retinal capillaries
- Outer barrier: tight junctions of the pigment epithelium

Fluorescein angiography makes it possible to locate the alterations of the blood-retina barrier, which can be subdivided into two parts.

- Inner blood-retina barrier: Retinal capillaries, located in the superficial layers of the retina have an endothelium whose cells, unlike the capillaries of other parts of the body, present tight junctions that make them watertight to fluorescence.

- Outer blood-retina barrier: The choriocapillaris lets the fluorescein seep freely from normal choroid so that it easily penetrates into the surrounding tissues, but it is blocked by the cells of the pigment epithelium. Also these cells are held by tight junctions that prevent the diffusion of the molecules towards the retina.

Consequently, at the level of the normal retinal capillaries, fluorescein is confined within the vessels enabling them to be perfectly visualized. In the choriocapillaris, the fluorescein that leaks out easily from the vessels is masked and its diffusion is blocked by the presence of the normal pigment epithelium screen.

Alterations in the blood-retina barrier produce a diffuse leakage hyperfluorescence, and secondarily pooling of the dye or tissue staining. These lesions may be located both in the inner barrier (endothelium of the capillaries) and in the outer barrier (pigment epithelium). These phenomena, due to leaks in the blood-retina barrier, increase in the later phases, more appropriately called tissue phase.

As example, let us mention the leakage dot of the central serous chorioretinopathy. This hyperfluorescent spot is located in the altered pigment epithelium (external blood-retina barrier) whose cells let diffuse the fluorescein in a very small area.

The reasons for this syndrome are still being debated: some authors consider it to be due to a focal pigment epithelium primitive lesion with tight junctions alteration, others attribute it to a vascular disorder in the underlying choriocapillaris.

Lesions of the retinal capillaries (inner blood-retina barrier), for example in diabetic retinopathy, clinically lead to the appearance of localized or diffuse retinal edema, exudates, cystoid edema and, in the more severe cases, hemorrhages. The fluorescein angiographic aspect is again leakage followed by pooling and tissue staining.

Fluorophotometry may quantify the alterations of the blood-retina barrier. A complex optic device, connected to a computer, makes it possible to track the fluorescence levels of the vitreous and of the other eye tissues and compare the results with other cases and various disorders. The results are very interesting but this technique is not widely used in clinical examination. It allows to measure the action of various drugs on the alterations of the blood-retina barrier.

PART IV

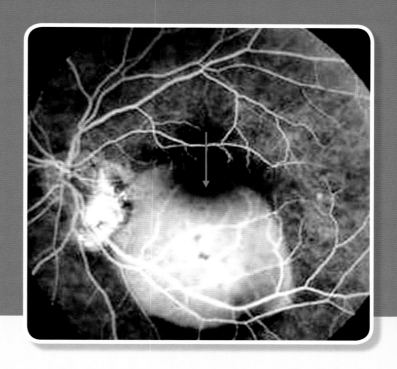

Pathological Fluorescein Angiography-Synthesis

Synthetic Evaluation

SYNTHESIS AND DEDUCTION

Synthesis is the last and most important step of an analysis process, completing the logical analytic method. It assesses globally all the data obtained from the various examinations carried out on the patient and allows the deduction of the diagnosis. This process involves both a technical dimension and an intellectual aspect and is the final and most important part of an analysis procedure. This mandatory step should not be bypassed by a hasty attempt to jump at a conclusion.

Diagnosis is too important to be guessed and should be the logical conclusion of a methodology. Diagnosis can be easy and quick or necessitate a long reflection and meditation.

The deductive and synthetic study is the most important final stage of ocular imaging interpretation, when using the method of logic deductive reasoning we are trying to teach in this handbook. *It implies, if too hasty, important risks of error.*

Synthesis consists in a global evaluation of the data obtained from the qualitative and quantitative analysis of fluorescein angiography, from the clinical history, clinical examination, the indocyanine green angiographic studies, autofluorescence not forgetting microperimetry that brings functional information. Cross section and en face OCT imaging present us today with a huge quantity of data we have to assess. It is now an integral part of fluorescein angiography assessing process.

The retina specialist who interprets the fluorescein angiography must be able to rely on a series of other data as well: age of the patient, visual acuity, history of the disease, general history of the patient, cardiovascular examination, etc. These elements make it possible to truly understand and evaluate the angiogram and not just "guess", as unfortunately some do.

In the first chapters we have separately highlighted the various alterations that fluorescein angiography may reveal: such alterations may be static (hyperfluorescence and hypofluorescence) or dynamic (filling rate, prolonged fluorescence, etc.). Indeed, in general, the fluorescein angiography alterations are associated in a very irregular fashion and they change during the different phases of the fluorescein angiography.

A synthetic evaluation of the fluorescein angiography requires not only a sound analytic knowledge of the abnormal elements of each frame but also the accurate study of the various fluorescein angiographic phases, paying special attention to the later phases that are very important; a complete series of all the frames is indispensable.

Also color photographs of the fundus, red-free light, fundus autofluorescence are indispensable, and where available can provide essential information.

Besides, it is also important to make a full study of the frames themselves. In some cases, as we shall see, it is mandatory to obtain a full topographic reconstruction of the retina. after the retina specialist acts as the cartographer who, after studying separately the maps of various towns and surroundings joins them together to obtain a representation of the whole country.

When the individual elements are combined together they take on a different meaning and enable an overall assessment of the ocular disorder (from the topographic standpoint and involvement of the various tissues and membranes of the eye). The isolated study of individual frames cannot provide such precise and comprehensive information.

It is the synthetic study of the fluorescein angiography that has made it possible in recent years to widen our knowledge about ocular disorders bringing up and making evident pathologic conditions that were not recognized in the past.

FLUORESCEIN ANGIOGRAPHY ASSESSMENT

We have to confront all the fluorescein angiography elementary lesions. During the analytical step we have broken down the fluorescein angiography in its various components.

Fluorescein angiography will be broken down, classified, reorganized, (including the qualitative elements, hyper- and hypofluorescence, as well as the morphological factors, the structure, architecture of retina. It is also essential to locate anatomically the seat of the abnormalities in the deeper and superficial layers).

The analysis is frequently made more difficult when the alterations are associated in a highly irregular way. Most of the operators in everyday work use only a small part of fluorescein angiography possibilities.

CLINICAL DATA NOT DIRECTLY RELATED TO FLUORESCEIN ANGIOGRAPHY

Clinical data not directly related to fluorescein angiography play an important part in the global evaluation of the case under study. Fluorescein angiography cannot be analyzed and assessed if we ignore the global aspect of the disease. The analyst must also have access to other information: patient's age and the general medical history, the results of a cardiovascular examination, and vision and ocular medical history, the progress of the disease, etc. He needs to be informed of the case history.

Most important is a complete ocular examination, including a slit lamp examination; the availability of photographs of the fundus and autofluorescence, the availability of an indocyanine green angiography; cross section and "en face" OCT, an echography, visual field, microperimetry, eye pressure, etc. It is essential to study all of the different phases of the fluorescein angiograms, from the first to the late stages. Here also he will analyze the various elements of a complete ocular examination.

Cross section and en face OCT imaging is now an important part of fluorescein angiography assessing process. Sometimes OCT imaging is used by some operators instead of fluorescein angiography.

SYNTHESIS PROCESS AND DEDUCTION

We begin by subdividing our data, and then we will put them together, classify, class, group, reorganize them, unite the elementary parts to form a few combined compounds.

The analytical steps must be complemented by the synthetic study of the angiograms. Synthesis process allows a global assessment of all the information obtained from the various examinations carried out on the patient and hence make a diagnosis. We will combine the various elements and parts to reconstruct a coherent complex.

The deduction step is the final part of the synthesis process, when we evaluate our organized and rearranged elements to draw inferences, come to a conclusion, arrive finally to a diagnosis. The accurate assessment of each of the basic elementary components of the fluorescein angiography analyzed allows to reach an exact diagnosis founded on logic.

DIFFICULTIES AND RISKS OF SYNTHESIS

The isolated study of the fluorescein angiography cannot provide an accurate and comprehensive information and does not permit to assess exactly the disorder. It should be recalled that in certain cases, a normal *fluorescein angiography* may correspond to an anomalous ocular fundus, and an apparently normal ocular fundus can correspond to an anomalous *fluorescein angiography. The disparate elements, when associated with one another, take on a different meaning, and allow the ocular disease to be considered from an all-encompassing perspective.* The study of all these images make it possible a comprehensive overall study of the patient's pathology.

Another risk of synthesis process is that in everyday practice we have to decide what data to preserve and what to *discard*. As a matter of fact, it is impossible to take always in account all the data. The big risk is, to unwittingly discard important elements. We are obliged to ignore an important quantity of information not to be overwhelmed by it, and we risk, doing so, to miss important facts and figures.

We risk also not to be perfectly balanced in our assessment and to do not give due importance to some useful information and to give too much attention to secondary facts.

And thus the last stage of the analytical process reorganizes, rearranges, recombines all the different data to arrive to a diagnosis by deductive reasoning, and to decide the treatment.

Summing up, the synthetic study of *fluorescein angiography* has made it possible to understand previously poorly known pathological conditions, to expand the horizons of knowledge about ocular diseases. *Fluorescein angiography* has led in the first years to important discoveries about the fundus disorders. It has changed the understanding of retinal diseases and their evolution. The synthetic study of fluorescein angiography has enabled to identify the triangular lesions of the choroid and the other

breakdowns of the circulation of the choroid, to describe and explain the "drop-shaped" or gravitational alterations of the epithelium to recognize the various types of proliferating diabetic retinopathy.

Recently, in the last 10 years, the introduction of time domain, then of spectral domain OCT, has allowed enrichments in the understanding of *fluorescein angiography*.

We believe that one of the most important fields in the future of fluorescein angiography will be connected to cross section and en face OCT and consist of the evaluation of new therapeutic treatments, including new intravitreal, subretinal injections, new retrobulbar treatments and therapeutic intravitreal implants, etc.

In the foreseeable future, we will certainly have new **angiography devices based on en face OCT** allowing angiography without dye and without invasive practice, using new wavelengths that will be even better, in terms of examination, depth penetration, speed, precision, and accuracy. Already **angiography devices based on en face OCT** allow studies of retinal and optic disc circulation. Some OCT angiography devices will study retinal physiology and, probably, semi-automated OCT angiography diagnosis will soon appear in ophthalmology to help the overworked retina specialist.

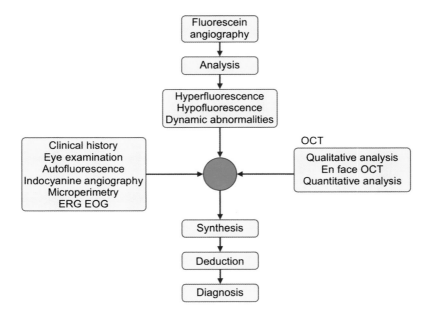

PART V

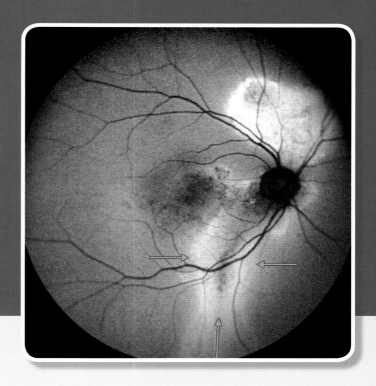

Major Fluorescein Angiography Syndromes

The fifth section of this book examines the major fluorescein angiography syndromes. These cases are most difficult due to images complexity in which the hypofluorescence or hyperfluorescence is not due to a single cause but to an intrication of diagnostic elements that need to be identified, compared and associated with various syndromes.

The fluorescein angiographies that are examined in the following chapters present various types of hyperfluorescence and hypofluorescence in more or less complex combinations. Our aim is to insist on the fact that each syndrome must be identified essentially on the basis of an *analytic study* of the data, which is then followed by a *synthesis* of all the heterogeneous elements to make a diagnosis. This fluorescein angiographic diagnosis is necessary in order to make a prognosis and prescribe a therapy.

CHAPTER 10

Diabetic Retinopathy

Retinal fluorescein angiography, OCT, laser photoco-agulation and intravitreal antiangiogenic treatments have modified and improved the knowledge of diabetic retinopathy and its prognosis.

Diabetic retinopathy develops in nearly all patients with long-standing diabetes. Clinically it is subdivided into proliferative and non-proliferative retinopathy.

Fluorescein angiography must be used in all diabetic patients, even if there are no retinal lesions, when the disease has been present for more than 8 years and in patients in whom, even if the disease has been present for a shorter time there are fundus signs of diabetic retinopathy. Fluorescein angiography must then be repeated every year or every 6 months and even more frequently if treatment is provided.

Retinal fluorescein angiography is mandatory when studying diabetic retinopathy, its evolution, its prognosis and its treatment follow-up. Indeed, used along OCT, it allows to:

- Analyze retinal abnormalities and assess their degree of severity;
- Determine the cause of visual loss;
- Specify the retinal situation at any given moment and track its evolution;
- Assess the risk of retinal edema and of neovascularization
- Decide whether and what treatment is needed;
- Locate the areas that require treatment;
- Check the efficacy of treatment.
- Follow evolution of the disease.

Optical coherence tomography (OCT) is also important in the assessment follow-up and treatment of diabetic retinopathy, for the evaluation and quantification of retinal edema, of the thickness and volume of the retina, for deciding the need for Laser and intravitreal treatment and post treatment monitoring.

It is superior in the diagnosis of macular edema to fluorescein angiography, but does not allow to see the ischemic lesions.

CLASSIFICATION

Among classifications, the very complex Airlie House classification was for 40 years most widely used in research and in studies on diabetes. Many other classifications of more practical interest have been used. A simpler and clinically useful one was for many years Zweng and Little's classification.

At **the 2002 American Academy of Ophthalmology meeting a new classification was adopted**, that is now used all over the world. This classification includes five levels:

1. No diabetic retinopathy,
2. Mild non-proliferative diabetic retinopathy (NPDR),
3. Moderate non-proliferative diabetic retinopathy (NPDR),
4. Severe non-proliferative diabetic retinopathy (NPDR),
5. Proliferative diabetic retinopathy (PDR).

Mild non-proliferative diabetic retinopathy shows only microaneurysms.

Moderate non-proliferative diabetic retinopathy is between mild and severe NPDR.

Severe non-proliferative diabetic retinopathy is based on the ETDRS. The specialist divides the fundus into four quadrants centered on the optic nerve and controls the quadrants with slit-lamp. If hemorrhages are present in all four quadrants or there is venous beading, severe NPDR is present. If one or more quadrant has intraretinal microvascular abnormalities (IRMAs), severe NPDR is present.

As the level of ischemia increases, **proliferative diabetic retinopathy** develops. In it, we find all the alterations listed above in addition to neovascular proliferation. Neovascular proliferation may be seen at the disc (neovascularization of the disc [NVD]) or at the edge of ischemic retinal areas (neovascularization elsewhere [NVE]). Tangential and anterioposterior vitreoretinal traction causes vitreous hemorrhages and tractional retinal detachment.

In addition, the **presence or absence of diabetic macular edema** is classified apart.

When edema is present, there are three possibilities:
1. Edema is far from the center (mild DME).
2. Edema is close to the center (moderate DME)
3. Edema involves the center (severe DME).

Diabetic macular edema (be focal or diffuse) may be observed at any stage of DR.

In focal edema, usually a ring of hard exudates surrounds microaneurysms and IRMA.

In diffuse type, there are few exudates or microaneurysms.

In a small number of eyes, one may observe a vitreoretinal interface syndrome with vitreomacular traction.

For everyday clinical work, diabetic retinopathy may be more simply divided into proliferative and non-proliferative. A pre-proliferative situation is possible. It is essential to understand the *natural evolution* of the disease in order to prevent its complications. In incipient diabetic retinopathy, often mixed forms of exudative and ischemic capillary lesions are observed.

The exudative forms generally remain in the sphere of non-proliferative diabetic retinopathy that accounts for almost 90% of diabetic retinopathies. In these cases, evolution leads to severe macular exudative lesions that lead finally to legal blindness.

The ischemic forms instead may lead to proliferative retinopathies (about 10% of cases) whose normal evolution is towards hemorrhages, glial proliferation, retinal detachment, vascular glaucoma, painful blindness.

NON-PROLIFERATIVE DIABETIC RETINOPATHY

Underlying non-proliferative diabetic retinopathy are abnormalities of the capillaries that may be both capillary occlusions with non-perfused areas and capillary dilatations with leakage of the fluorescein; this leakage is due to an alteration in the endothelial cells junctions which is probably the first pathologic event underlying retinopathy. The onset of retinal lesions is generally related to the duration of the diabetic disease and is facilitated by an imperfect metabolic control (Figs 1 and 2A).

Angiographic Lesions of Capillaries

Fluorescence angiography highlights the following alterations:
- Dilated and irregular capillaries
- Increased wall permeability
- More evident and coarse capillary network of the macula
- Widening of the avascular area of the macula with, at times, interruptions in the capillary arcade
- Capillary micro-occlusions
- Microaneurysms.

Capillary Dilatations

This is the earliest and still reversible fluorescein angiographic sign. The capillaries are much more evident than in the fluorescein angiography of a normal retina and this is probably due to the occlusion of some capillaries and to the dilatation of others. In more advanced cases. Some capillary segments are dilated and tortuous and may simulate new formed vessels.

The avascular area of the fovea, that is normally about 500 microns is larger. The altered capillaries show some leaking of the fluorescein through their walls.

Ischemic Capillary Lesions—Retinal Hypoxia

The alterations of the retinal arterioles generally lead to ischemic alterations and evident fluorescein angiographic lesions. The fluorescein angiographies highlight very thin arterial capillaries. Often from an almost normal arteriole stems an arteriolar branch that is interrupted abruptly at the center or on the edges of a non-perfused retina area. At the level of these ischemic areas, ophthalmoscopy may often highlight cotton-wool exudates, while at the edges there may be venous alterations that take the form of irregular dilatations. Often there are rounded hemorrhages (located in the deeper retinal layers). Even more frequently found are clusters of microaneurysms at the periphery of the ischemic areas. The walls of the arterioles that cross ischemic areas are strongly stained by the dye (Fig. 3).

Microaneurysms

Microaneurysms are an early ophthalmoscopy lesion. Fluorescein angiography can highlight their onset in relationship with arteriolar micro-occlusions. They may be isolated or form clusters and often, if fluid is spreading through the altered walls, they may cause retinal edema and later actual exudates. Microaneurysms may increase, disappear in a given point and then reappear in other places.

Microaneurysms may be subdivided depending on their developmental stage.

Incipient microaneurysms are small, difficult to spot through ophthalmoscopy but clearly be seen through fluorescein angiography; fluorescein does not leak out through their walls.

Developed microaneurysms can be seen by ophthalmoscopy and fluorescein angiography; fluorescein leaks through their walls.

More developed microaneurysms vary in size, at times they are yellow at the ophthalmoscope with slightly irregular walls and marked leakage of fluorescein.

The last degree of evolution is towards atrophy. The thrombosed microaneurysm does not fill with dye. Some authors deem that microaneurysms are actually the abortive beginning of a neovascularization.

Intraretinal Microvascular Abnormalities (IRMA)

Dilated, tortuous capillary segments are often noticed in fluorangiographies that may mimic new formed vessels. These pathological aspects are generally visible where the capillary network is sparser. These lesions are intraretinal and some authors consider them to be the beginning of an intraretinal neovascularization whereas other authors think that these are only the localized lesions of pre-existing capillaries.

In any case, these abnormal dilated and tortuous vessels have altered walls with marked leakage of the fluorescein but they never lead to vitreous hemorrhages. Areas of retinal edema are frequently surrounded with hard exudates of lipoproteins deposited at their periphery forming a ring or a crown around the central lesions (Fig. 6).

Perimacular Capillary Network Alterations

In the early stages of diabetic retinopathy, changes in the macular capillary network show it more evident than in normal macula. This appearance is due to an increase in the size of some capillaries while others are closed and thus form a coarser network with larger and more sparse meshwork; there is also an evident increase in the size of the avascular area of the fovea. When ischemic areas are present, as frequently happens on the temporal side of the macula, the situation may evolve towards an interruption of the capillary arcades. The dye may leak from the altered vessels (Figs 2B to 2D).

Hard Exudates

Hard exudates that are evident at the ophthalmoscope are almost invisible with fluorescein angiography. However, when they are very thick and dense, their images provide imperfect masking. They consist of lipoproteins that precipitate at the boundary between the edematous and healthy retina; they are located in the deep layers of the retina; often they appear at a distance and around the vascular intraretinal abnormalities from which the edema expands. The hard exudates may be circinnate (form ring) or star-shaped. They often evolve into fibrous macular plaques with a severe impact on the visual function.

Quantification

Fluorescein angiography does not allow to map retinal edema. The OCT map is important for localizing focal edema, delimiting diffuse edema and showing

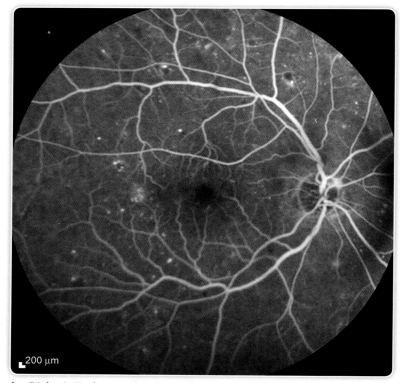

200 µm

Figure 1: Diabetic Retinopathy. Diabetic Background Retinopathy.

Capillary dilatations are the earliest and still reversible fluorescein angiographic sign. The capillaries are much more evident than in the fluorescein angiography of a normal retina and this is probably due to the occlusion of some capillaries and to the dilatation of others. The avascular area of the fovea, that is normally around 500 microns, is found to be larger. The altered capillaries may show some leaking of the fluorescein through their walls.

Alterations of the macular capillary network: In the early stages of diabetic retinopathy there are changes in the macular capillary network that is more evident than in normal conditions.

Arteriolar capillary lesions—retinal hypoxia. Some ischemic areas may be seen. The walls of the arterioles that pass through the ischemic areas are strongly stained by the dye.

Microaneurysms are the earliest seen lesions. Microaneurysms may increase, disappear in a given point and then reappear in other places. Incipient microaneurysms are small, but they can clearly be seen through fluorescein angiography; fluorescein may leak through their walls. Developed microaneurysms are bigger; fluorescein leaks out through their walls. Some microaneurysm clusters leaking dye may be seen.

edematous areas. Measuring retinal thickness and volume allows us to quantify edema, which enables us to decide when to treat and track the efficacy of therapy. There is a roughly inverse relationship between visual acuity and retinal thickness. As retinal thickness increases, visual acuity decreases, with or without the presence of cystoid edema. Measuring the retina's thickness and volume is essential for determining prognosis, assessing indications for surgery and monitoring disease progression.

Evolution

When there is a worsening of the areas of non-perfusion, they become more extensive as new capillary districts get occluded. Large areas become totally ischemic

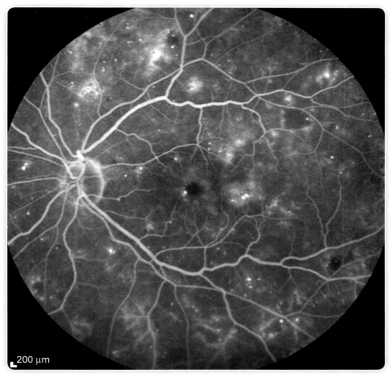

200 μm

Figure 2A: Diabetic Retinopathy. Non-proliferative Diabetic Retinopathy. The capillaries are much more evident than in the fluorescein angiography of a normal retina and this is probably due to the occlusion of some capillaries and to the dilatation of others. The avascular area of the fovea is enlarged and irregular in this case of diabetic retinopathy. The ischemic area is less fluorescent than the normal retina and is more easily viewed through contrast; along its borders there are dilated capillaries that form artero-venous anastomoses. Rare round hemorrhages are located in the deeper retinal layers. The capillaries that pass through the ischemic areas are strongly stained by the dye.

Microaneurysms may be seen isolated or in clusters and often, leaking through the altered walls, they may cause the onset of a retinal edema and later actual exudates. In many of them fluorescein leaks out through the walls. Developed microaneurysms are bigger; intraretinal microvascular anomalies are seen.

and, on the edges of these zones, the capillaries are abnormal, dilated, with frequent arteriovenous shunts; intraretinal microvascular abnormalities that seen in the fluorescein angiography increase in number and size. These abnormal but not new formed capillaries allow fluorescein to leak. We can also observe venous abnormalities with sausage shaped dilatation, venous loops and duplications (Fig. 4).

Fluorescein angiography highlights extensive ischemic areas whose localization is particularly frequent in the *mid-periphery*, especially in the inferior nasal quadrant. To the temporal side of the macula the areas of non-perfusion of the mid-periphery merge with the paramacular capillary exclusions causing at times an interruption in the arcade. There are often small deposits indicative of hard exudates, and microcavities of cystoid edema, hard and cotton wool exudates. The ischemic forms include closure of capillaries and proliferation of new vessels on the disc, retina, iris.

It is therefore very important to perform a **full fluorescein angiography extended to include the periphery and reconstruct the entire middle and far periphery of the retina through the device software, or a collage of frames**. The large ischemic areas determine

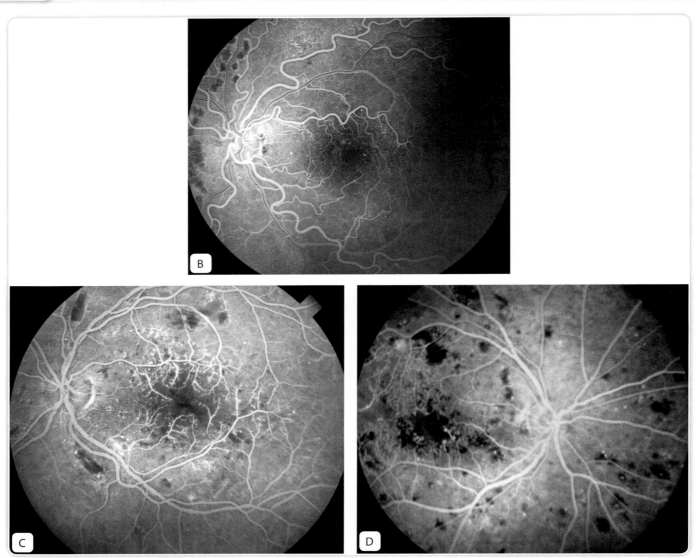

Figures 2B to D: Diabetic Retinopathy. Enlarged Avascular Area. The avascular area of the fovea, that is normally around 500 microns is enlarged in diabetic retinopathy. In the early stages of diabetic retinopathy, there are changes in the macular capillary network that is more evident than in normal conditions. This appearance is due to an increase in the size of some capillaries while others are closed and thus form a coarser network with larger and more sparse meshes; there is also an increase in the size of the avascular area of the fovea.

(B) When ischemic areas are present, the situation may evolve towards an interruption of the capillary arcades with marked decrease of visual acuity.

(C and D) The dye may leak from the altered vessels. Deep and superficial hemorrhages are seen.

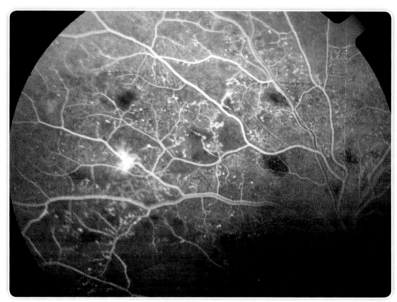

Figure 3: Diabetic Retinopathy. Non-perfused Areas. Ischemic alterations are seen in fluorescein angiographic lesions. The ischemic area is less fluorescent than the normal retina and is more easily seen through contrast with the surrounding healthy zones; along its borders are dilated capillaries that form artero-venous anastomoses. Hypofluorescence is observed in the capillary phase and is generally maintained in the subsequent phases. The fluorangiographies highlight very thin arterial capillaries. Often from an almost normal arteriole there stems an arteriolar branch that is interrupted abruptly at the center or on the edges of an ischemic area of the retina. Rare roundish hemorrhages (located in the deeper retinal layers) can be seen as some clusters of microaneurysms at the periphery of the ischemic areas. The walls of the arterioles that pass through the ischemic areas are strongly stained by the dye.

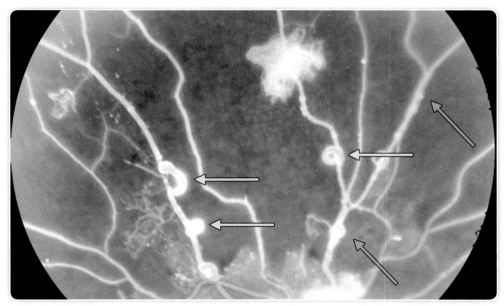

Figure 4: Diabetic Retinopathy—Venous Anomalies. These are anomalous dilated capillaries whose walls are strongly stained are seen in a non-perfused retinal district. There are also evident venous anomalies with moniliform, sausage like dilatation (arrows), venous loops (yellow arrows), and duplications. They are well seen on the darker background of the non-perfused retina.

the production of a vascular proliferation factor and the new vessels generally grow at the periphery of these non-perfused areas.

It is useful to recognize this stage of the diabetic retinopathy that precedes the onset of neoformed vessels. It is still being discussed whether the extended areas of ischemia should be treated with photocoagulation or wait for the onset of the first hemorrhages. It may be prudent to perform preventive photocoagulation of the ischemic areas and of the surrounding microvascular alterations.

Evolution of non-proliferative retinopathy leads to worsening of cystoid edema and later to a fibrous central scar.

Patients presenting with diabetic macular edema have currently many treatment possibilities: grid laser photocoagulation, intravitreal anti-angiogenic drugs and intravitreal cortisone implants. Fluorescein angiography and OCT are mandatory in determining the optimal ophthalmic therapy and in following the progression of the disease.

Ischemic Vascular Alterations Leading to Proliferative Retinopathy

After a few years, evolution ischemic vascular alterations can appear and progress to retinal capillary non-perfusion, resulting in a clinical picture of the retina characterized by increased numbers of hemorrhages, venous abnormalities, and intraretinal microvascular abnormalities.

It will lead over time frequently to proliferative retinopathy with retinal detachment, vascular glaucoma, and blindness.

The OCT shows in the retinal ischemic areas thickened *inner layers of the retina* with a spongy type of edema.

DIABETIC MACULOPATHY

Macular edema is the leading cause of visual impairment in non-proliferative diabetic retinopathy.

Table 1: Diabetic maculopathies
Maculopathy with focal edema
Maculopathy with diffuse edema
Maculopathy with cystoid edema
Macular serous elevation of the retina
Ischemic maculopathy
Traction maculopathy

It starts with focal edema and progresses toward diffuse retinal edema. OCT is more useful than fluorescein angiography to detect areas of thickened and hyporeflective spongy retina.

Focal and Diffuse Edema

In diffuse or localized retinal edema, the fluorescein spreads from the vascular walls, staining the retinal tissue without any pooling of the dye. The starting point may be a diffuse vascular alteration, as occurs in diabetic microangiopathy.

Focal edema is more easily detected with OCT than with fluorescein angiography. It shows a thickened, spongy retina. It is hyporeflective with decreased optical backscattering. The OCT retinal map is important in cases of focal edema, because it allows better localization than fluorescein angiography to decide treatment. Laser, it also helps confirm treatment efficacy. Viewed with OCT, the retina is thickened and shows numerous tiny, irregular cavities that resemble spongy tissue. The areas of low reflectivity are increased, but above all, evident in *the outer retinal layers*. Edematous areas are hyporeflective with decreased optical backscattering. *Outer retinal layers* are the preferred locations of diabetic edema. The outer plexiform layer shows the most edema. It is believed that the areas of spongy retina in the OCT highlight altered Müller cells. After years of progression of diffuse edema, the irregular micro spaces merge, resulting in the first pseudocysts.

Cystoid Macular Edema

Persistent retinal edema results in necrosis of the Müller cells, leading cystoid cavity formation in the retina.

These spaces start in the outer plexiform layer, and subsequently penetrate the nuclear layers and the inner plexiform layer. Advanced cystoid edema permeates the retina, bringing residual tissue to atrophy. Fluorescein angiographically, the cavities of the cystoid macular edema form a screen against the normal fluorescence in the earlier phases, and then pooling spots appear issuing from the posterior pole capillaries. In the later phases, the aspect is typical with the hyperfluorescent pseudocystic cavities flower shaped around the foveal area.

Cystoid edema remains highly hyperfluorescent even in the later phases up to one or two hours from the beginning of the fluorescein examination. At this point the pseudocysts have blurred edges with slight dye leakage (Fig. 5).

It is important to quantify the edema by measuring its volume as well as retina thickness and the surface of the cystoid lesions. Edema topography is important to know to foresee the retinopathy development.

In cystoid macular edema, we observe chronic pooling of intraretinal fluid in pseudocystic formations or intraretinal cavities arranged around the fovea. Its aspect has been likened to the petals of a flower or honeycomb. Initially the fovea is not involved. However, later, a central loggia may appear that entails a marked and final decrease in the vision.

Serous Detachment

Serous detachment in diabetic retinopathy is not seen with fluorescein angiography. Optical coherence tomography has shown that serous detachments are

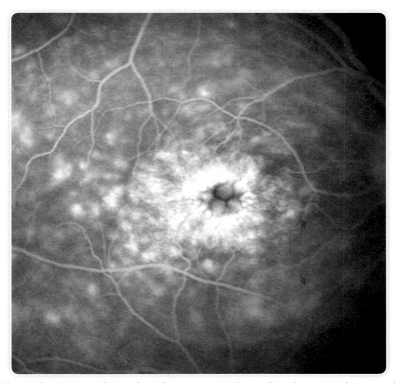

Figure 5: Diabetic Retinopathy. Diabetic Cystoid Macular Edema. In cystoid macular edema, we observe a chronic pooling of intraretinal fluid in pseudocystic formations arranged around the fovea. They may look as the flower petals. During the evolution central cysts may appear that entail a sharp decrease in the visual acuity. Fluorescein angiographically, the microcysts of the cystoid macular edema form a screen against the normal fluorescence in the earlier phases, and then dye pools in the cavities. Some leakage spots appear starting from the capillaries of the posterior pole. The cystoid edema remains very hyperfluorescent even in the late fluorescein angiography phases.

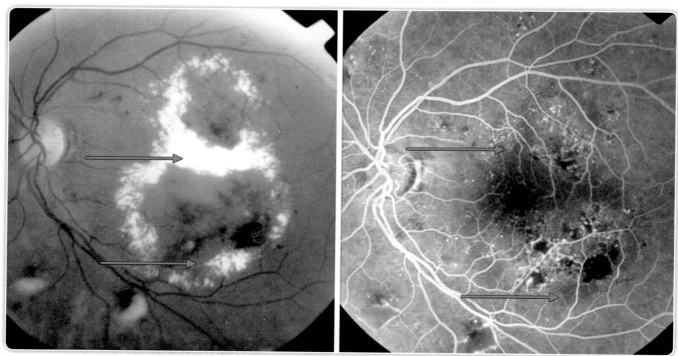

Figure 6: Diabetic Retinopathy IRMA and Circinate Exudates. During evolution of the diabetic retinopathy there is an increase in the intraretinal microvascular anomalies (IRMA) that appear in the fluorescein angiography. Dilated, tortuous capillary segments may simulate new formed vessels. These pathological aspects are generally visible where the capillary network is more sparse. The anomalous dilated and tortuous vessels have altered walls with marked leakage of the fluorescein. They produce edema but they never lead to hemorrhages of the vitreous. Retinal edema is frequently found with hard exudates of lipoproteins deposited at their periphery forming a crown around the central lesion (circinate exudates). Hard exudates form a screen in the early phases of the fluorescein angiography, but then the screen decreases and becomes incomplete (arrows).

part of the final progression of diabetic edema. A small localized serous retinal detachment with optically blank cavity between the detached retina and the pigment epithelium can be seen. Serous detachment is less frequent than diffuse edema or cystoid edema.

Traction edema is seen when the tension applied by epiretinal membrane leads to retraction of the inner limiting membrane. In these cases of traction, edema the fluorescein spreads from the vascular walls, staining the retinal tissue. In a few cases, some pooling of the dye can be seen. The starting point is traction on retina, but there is also a diffuse vascular alteration.

The OCT enables us to detect epiretinal membranes. At times, these are easily differentiated, but sometimes they merge with the retinal nerve fiber layer. This membrane, with its tractions on the retina, causes edema, retinal folds and sometimes serous detachments.

Ischemic Maculopathy

Ischemic maculopathy at onset shows small alteration in the macular capillary arcade. There is an increase in the size of some capillaries while others are closed and thus we see a coarser network with larger and sparse meshwork; the increase in the size of the avascular area of the fovea is evident.

When ischemic areas are present on the temporal side of the macula, the situation may evolve towards an important interruption of the capillary arcades.

Peripheral non-perfused zones merge with the enlarged ischemic avascular macular area. The dye may leak from the altered vessels. No treatment is possible.

PROLIFERATIVE RETINOPATHY

Proliferative retinopathy is most frequent among young people: it may be a developmental stage of non-proliferative retinopathy or it may appear early: new vessels appear that are initially preretinal and then prepapillary and intravitreal. These neovascularization is formed by capillaries with very fragile single cell walls and may cause vitreal hemorrhages with ensuing glial proliferation (Figs 7 to 9).

New Vessels

These new vessels generally appear at the edges of the ischemic areas; initially they can be recognized because they are very irregular and give rise to an intense leakage of the fluorescein. In the earlier phases of the fluorescein angiography, the branching and irregularity of the neovascular network is quite evident. The walls of the new vessels are made up of a single cell layer that is highly permeable to the fluorescein and is quite fragile. A few seconds after filling their net is masked by the intense diffusion of the fluorescein. Often preretinal hemorrhages or vitreous haze are quite evident caused by hemorrhages from the very fragile new vessels. Pan retinal (scatter) photocoagulation almost always produces a full regression of these vessels.

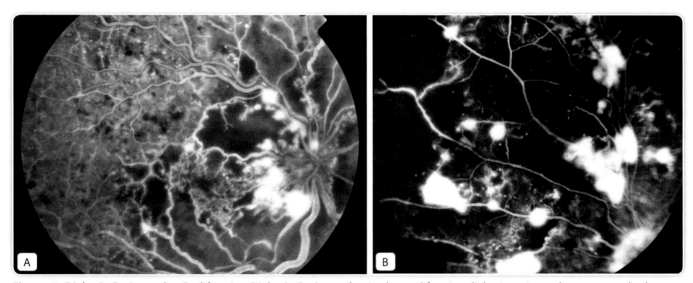

Figure 7: Diabetic Retinopathy. Proliferative Diabetic Retinopathy. In the proliferative diabetic retinopathy new vessels show an intense dye leakage. The new vessels appear on the edge of areas of non-perfusion. These areas become broader and more extensive as successive capillary districts get occluded, with more new vessels forming. The ischemia determines the production of a vascular proliferation. New formed capillaries are very thin, fragile and their walls leak easily fluorescein. These new vessels show an intense dye leakage. In the figure a few laser spots are seen.

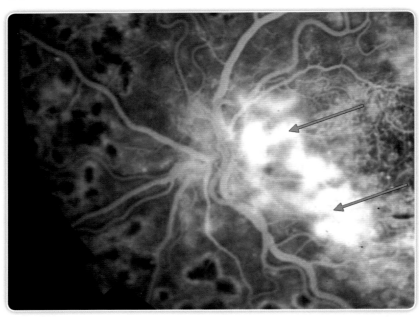

Figure 8: Diabetic Retinopathy. Proliferative Diabetic Retinopathy. New Vessels of the Retina and Optic Disc. In the proliferative diabetic retinopathy, new vessels appear on the edge of areas of non-perfusion. The ischemia determines vascular proliferation. New formed capillaries finally interest the optic disc with intense vascular proliferation from the papilla and retina (arrows) showing an intense leakage.

The *biggest risk factors for severe visual loss* in proliferative retinopathy are listed below:
- Vascular membrane of the disc larger than one quarter of the diameter of the capillary;
- New vessels of the optic papilla associated with hemorrhages;
- New preretinal vessels associated with preretinal or vitreous hemorrhages of one or more papilla diameters.

Proliferative retinopathy, untreated or treated too late, evolves towards vitreous hemorrhages that can initially regress, but if they occur again and again they will cause very severe conditions. Some consequences are glial proliferation of the new vessels with traction on the retina and retinal detachments that are initially localized and then become extensive, and finally neovascular glaucoma.

Proliferative retinopathy is the major indication for pan-retinal photocoagulation, which when performed early and correctly, provides very good results. Proliferative retinopathy is a bad prognostic factor for the life of the patient: 55% of affected individuals may die within 5 years from onset.

Table 2: Causes of preretinal and papillary neovascularization other than diabetic retinopathy: Extensive retinal ischemia

Frequent causes:
- Occlusions of the central retinal vein
- Occlusions of the venous branches
- Eales' disease
- Other vasculitis
- Pars planitis
- Sickle-cell anemia
- Thalassemia

Rare causes:
- Leukemia
- Cryoglobulinemia
- Waldenstrom disease
- Multiple myeloma
- Unknown causes

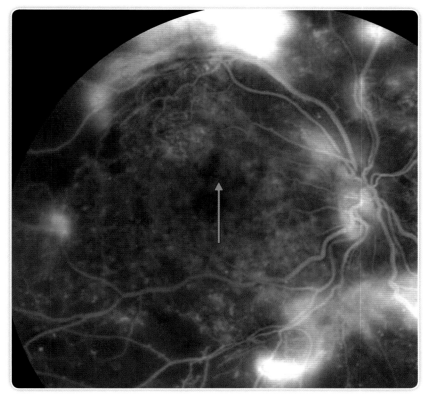

Figure 9: Diabetic Retinopathy. Proliferative Diabetic Retinopathy and Non-perfused Areas. Fluorescein angiography highlights extensive ischemic areas whose localization is particularly frequent in the mid-periphery, especially in the inferior nasal quadrant, as shown in this case. To the temporal side of the macula, the areas of non-perfusion of the mid-periphery merge with the paramacular capillary exclusions causing an interruption in the arcade (arrow).

It is therefore very important to perform a full fluorescein angiography extended to include the periphery and reconstruct the entire middle and far periphery of the retina through a collage of frames or automated reconstruction. The extended areas of ischemia determine the production of a vascular proliferation factor and the new vessels generally arise at the periphery of the same areas of non-perfusion. These new vessels show an intense dye leakage.

Age-related Macular Degeneration and Other Macular Degenerations

AGE-RELATED MACULAR DEGENERATION

Senile macular degeneration is one of the major causes for severe visual loss in the world. The disorder usually begins with drusen that may give rise to atrophic alterations or to subretinal new vessels.

- **Drusen**

  Colloid bodies or drusen are frequently found in the senile eye. They are degenerative formations of Bruch's membrane (not to be confused, at ophthalmoscopy, with hard exudates); they are roundish and yellowish, and are found mainly at the posterior pole. Histological examination subdivide them into *hard* drusen, small hyaline deposits with sharp boundaries, and *soft* drusen, deposits of granular material. As regards the pathogenesis, the most common theory is that it is the waste material deriving from the cells of degenerating pigment epithelium.

  The fluorescein angiographic aspect is *window effect* in the earlier phases and then *staining* of the lesion in the later phases; the staining is however less than that is seen for instance in the vascular walls of occluded vessels. The drusen may not evolve for years or they may undergo transformations with widening and merging and formation of calcium deposits.

  They may evolve into the *atrophic* form or towards *disciform* macular degeneration, but it is important to remember that only a minimal part of the drusen will lead to these complications.

  The OCT shows drusen as irregularities and undulations of the pigment epithelium. Contents are slightly hyper-reflective. It frequently possible to observe Bruch's membrane as a thin line. "En face" scans show clusters of roundish hollow formations (Figs 1 and 2).

- **Atrophic (dry) age-related macular degeneration**

  The macular region shows many drusen and a progressive atrophy of the pigment epithelium, of the external retinal layers and of the choriocapillaris. These alterations are evident in fluorescein angiography where the limit between the healthy and atrophic retina is quite sharp. This causes visual loss but the evolution is very slow and the patient will generally have a final visual acuity that is better than in the disciform type. Mention can be made of areolar or geographic atrophy, a clinical form described earlier when discussing the "window" defects (Fig. 4).

- **Serous (wet) age-related macular degeneration**

  In the typical form, various combinations are seen of serous elevation of the pigment epithelium, serous elevation of the retina, subepithelial and subretinal hemorrhages. The hemorrhages may infiltrate the entire retina and appear also at the surface. At the boundaries of the serous elevation some hard exudates may appear. The cause of the serous elevation and of the hemorrhages is the presence of a new vascular membrane (CNV) probably provoked by a damage to Bruch's membrane. The cluster of new vessels that are very thin, show evident leakage of the dye and appears first below the Retinal Pigment Epithelium and then penetrates into the subretinal space. The fluorescein angiography easily highlights the serous elevation of the retina with progressive pooling of the fluorescein and the hemorrhages whose depth is evidenced by the screen effect that they have on the fluorescence of retinal vessels, capillaries and choroid.

The neovascular membrane is generally quite evident at the beginning with a stalk at the center and a periphery like a "bicycle wheel" consisting of fine anastomoses of the new vessels (Figs 3A and B and 5).

Frequently instead, one can barely make out its presence, hidden as it is by the hemorrhages; there are also occult forms, located below the retinal pigment epithelium (Figs 6 to 9A to D).

- **Disciform age-related macular degeneration**
  After a long evolution and repeated treatments, disciform AMD shows various combinations of pigment deposits, glial tissue, serous elevation of the pigment epithelium, serous elevation of the retina, subepithelial and subretinal hemorrhages. At the edges of the serous detachments may appear hard exudates and cystoid edema. Hemorrhages may infiltrate the entire retina and then regress leaving glial scars (Figs 10A and B).

- **Pigment epithelium tears**
  The retinal pigment epithelium tear is a severe complication of age-related macular degeneration. It appears in the natural evolution of serous detachment or serous-hemorrhagic detachment of the pigment epithelium and heavily worsens its prognosis.

  It is frequently a complication of the intravitreal treatment of age-related macular degeneration.

  The rupture of the retinal pigment epithelium appears as a result of rip of the pigment epithelium on the margin of the serous detachment that is more distant from the foveal areas. It is located at the border between elevated epithelium and healthy epithelium. The pigment epithelium flap, free in the sub-retinal space, can behave in either of the two following ways:

1. It may roll up on as a papyrus roll
2. It remains gaping in the subretinal space and then retracts.

The successive adhesion of the edges onto Bruch's membrane will give rise to a serous detachment that might be called the "secondary" detachment (Figs 11A and B).

- **Fibrous disciform scar**
  Subretinal hemorrhages regress generally giving way to a fibrous disciform scar. The fibrous glial tissue infiltrates the subretinal neovascularization between the altered Bruch's membrane and the elevated retina. The scar surface also includes other hyperplastic elements of the pigment epithelium. The final scar is generally dry with deep destruction of all the tissues of the posterior pole. More rarely, it is accompanied by widespread exudates and elevation of the entire sensory retinal of the posterior pole. This detachment at times spreads at times, even beyond the vascular arcades.

AMD: Idiopathic Polypoidal Vasculopathy

About 10 to 20% of AMD patients are affected with an atypical form of macular disorder known as Idiopathic Polypoidal Vasculopathy. Fluorescein angiography shows angiomas associated with serous and hemorrhagic detachments of the retina and of the pigment epithelium (Figs 12A to D).

Indocyanine green angiography reveals a thin vascular network in the choroid layer, with cluster of polypoidal angiomas and serous and hemorrhagic detachments of the retina and of the pigment epithelium.

The OCT scans show small cup-shaped elevations of the pigment epithelium containing fibrovascular tissue in the cupola of the PED and serous and hemorrhagic detachments of the retina and pigment epithelium. Sometimes a stalk can be seen from the choroid to the vascular tissue in the RPE detachment.

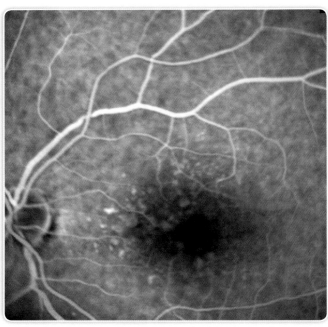

Figure 1: Macular Degeneration. Colloid Bodies or Soft Drusen. Colloid bodies or drusen are degenerative formations of Bruch's membrane; they are roundish and yellowish, and are found mainly in the posterior pole. *Soft* drusen are deposits of granular or amorphous material and measure more than 60 micron. The most common theory is that they are formed by degradation material deriving from the degenerating pigment epithelium cells. The fluorescein angiographic aspect is the *window effect* in the earlier phases and then *staining* of the lesion in the later phases. The drusen may remain unvaried for years or they may undergo transformations with widening and confluence and formation of calcium deposits. They may grow and merge together forming drusenoid detachments.

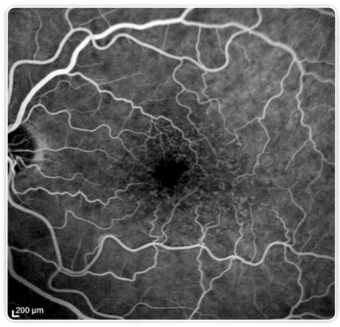

Figure 2: Macular Degeneration. Hard Drusen. Hard drusen are small hyaline deposits with sharp boundaries. They give a window effect in the earlier phases and then staining in the later phases. They measure less than 60 micron.

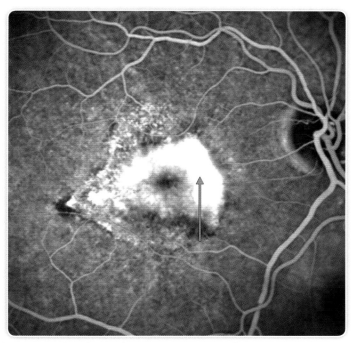

Figure 3A: Macular Degeneration. Age-related Macular Degeneration—Classic Neovascularization. Fluorescein Angiography.
A large hyperfluorescent (arrow) area shows classic neovascularization (CNV). Rare dark hemorrhages block the posterior layers fluorescence. Some pigment epithelium dystrophy surrounds the CNV.

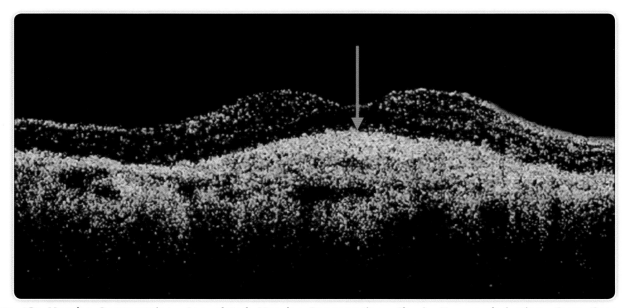

Figure 3B: Macular Degeneration. Age-related Macular Degeneration—Classic Neovascularization. Cross Scan OCT.
A large hyper-reflective area is seen under the retina (arrow): classic neovascularization is located above RPE.

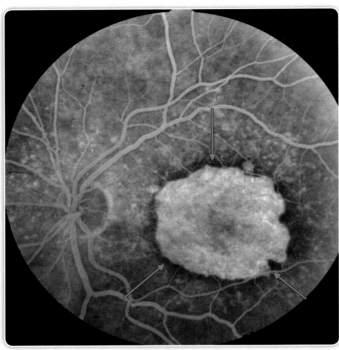

Figure 4: Macular Degeneration. AMD, Areolar Atrophy. Anomalous Transmission of Fluorescence. Window Defect. The fluorescein angiographic aspect is typical of a window defect. Hyperfluorescence begins in the choroidal phase and is well delimited by sharp margins (arrows) of the opening in the pigmented epithelium. The window here is rounded and does not overlap precisely to the alteration as seen with ophthalmoscopy.

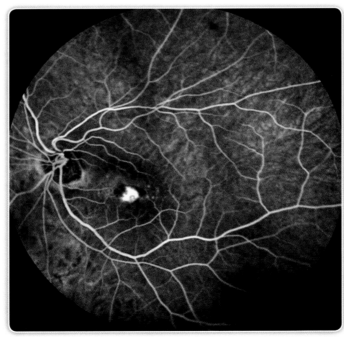

Figure 5: Macular Degeneration. AMD—Drusen and Classic Neovascularization. One hyperfluorescent area ringed with pigment deposits shows classic neovascularization. Some dark hemorrhages block the posterior layers fluorescence. Colloid bodies or drusen are found in this age-related macular degeneration.

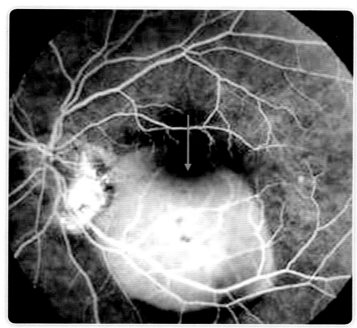

Figure 6: Macular Degeneration. AMD with Pigment Epithelium Detachment. A serous elevation of the pigment epithelium can be seen. It is hyperfluorescent but not homogenous. Dark hemorrhages showing an horizontal level block the inferior layers fluorescence. An occult neovascular membrane is probably located at the superior notch (arrow).

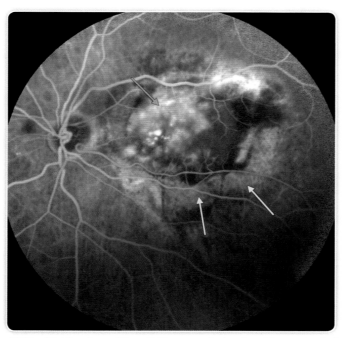

Figure 7: Macular Degeneration. AMD with Classic and Occult Neovascularization. The markedly hyperfluorescent areas correspond to classic neovascularization (arrow). A serous elevation of the pigment epithelium can be seen as well as serous detachment of the retina. Dark subepithelial and subretinal hemorrhages block the posterior layers fluorescence. The hemorrhages infiltrate the entire retina and appear also at the surface. Pigment deposits are found. At the boundaries of the elevation appear some hard exudates. On the degeneration inferior side tiny granulous hyperfluorescent dots can be seen (yellow arrow). These hyperfluorescent micro dots correspond to an occult membrane.

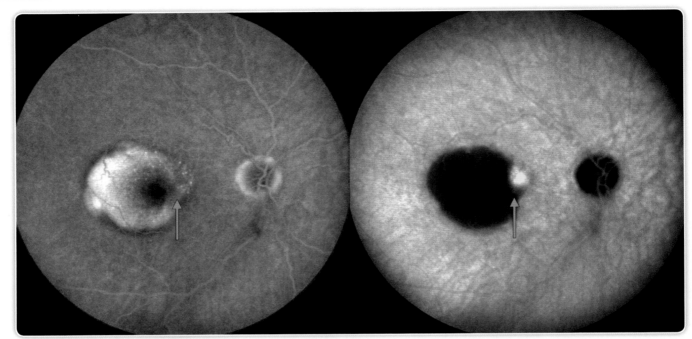

Figure 8: Macular Degeneration. AMD with Occult Neovascularization. In this case, we observe a pigment epithelium detachment on the fluorescein angiography in the figure at the left hand side. The pigment epithelium detachment is hyperfluorescent. On the PED right side some punctiform granulous hyperfluorescent dots can be seen (arrow). The ICG angiography (figure right hand side) shows these hyperfluorescent micro dots correspond to an occult membrane (arrow). Note that PED are black, hypofluorescent at ICG.

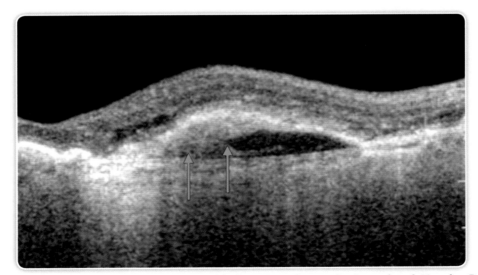

Figure 9I: Macular Degeneration. B-scan of Pigment Epithelium Detachment in Age-related Macular Degeneration. Cross sectional OCT scan show a vast pigment epithelium detachment. Some cystoid edema cells are seen close to PED in retina layers. PED contents are not homogenous. Inside the PED, close to cupola and on the left side of the detachment we see an hyper-reflective area relative to fibrovascular membrane (arrows). The outer retina is disrupted as well as IS/OS junction (ellipsoid).

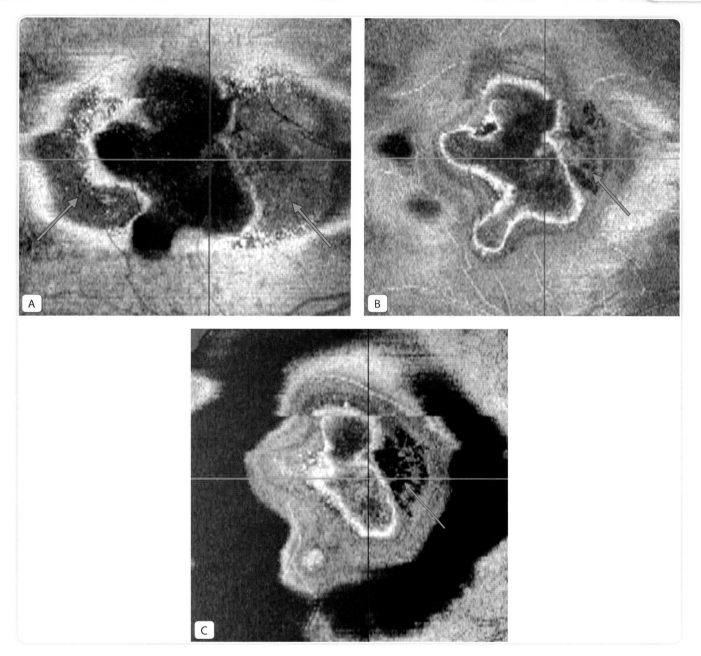

Figures 9IIA to C: Macular Degeneration. Pigment Epithelium Detachment in Age-related Macular Degeneration "En Face" OCT.
En Face OCT scans show that Pigment epithelium detachments in AMD have an irregular oval or multilobular aspects. In this case PED shape is multilobular. "en face" scans allow the study of pigment epithelium detachments walls that are found to be thick, granular (never smooth) and irregular.
We show here three "en face" scans (A, B, C) the **first section (A)** parallel to pigment epithelium is placed at RPE level, its contents are optically free. The **second section (B)** is placed half way up the detachment. The **third smaller scan (C)** contents are hyper- reflective, located at the cupola and show that vascular and fibrovascular tissue is adherent to the RPE detachment dome (yellow arrow). Outside the pigment epithelium detachment small dark areas of cystoid edema are seen (arrow)
PDE walls are granular and irregularly thick in some points and thin in other; they surround hyporeflective or slightly hyper-reflective areas corresponding to the contents of the serous detachments

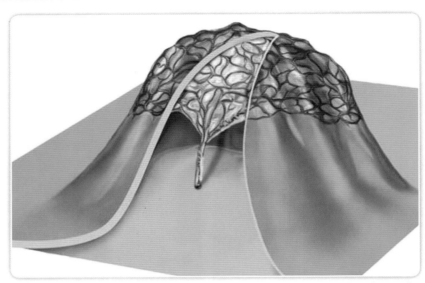

Figure 9D: Macular Degeneration. Drawing: Pigment Epithelium Detachment in Age-related Macular Degeneration "En Face" OCT. A color drawing summarize the normal appearance of pigment epithelium detachments in AMD and shows that vascular and fibrovascular tissue is adherent to the RPE detachment dome.

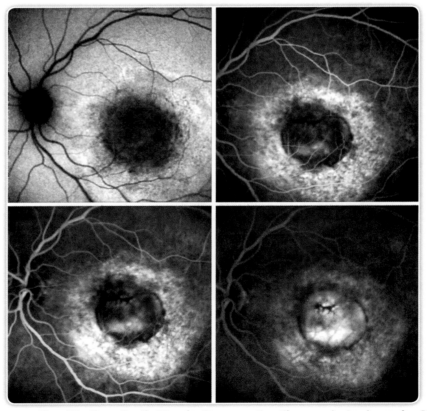

Figure 10A: Macular Degeneration. Disciform Senile Macular Degeneration Fluorescein Angiography. Disciform degeneration is the end result of a long evolution in non-treated AMD. We can see serous elevation of the pigment epithelium, serous detachment of the retina, subepithelial and subretinal hemorrhages, cystoid macular edema. The hemorrhages infiltrate the entire retina and appear also at the surface. Pigment deposits are always found. At the boundaries of the elevation appear some hard exudates. Later fibroglial tissue will develop.

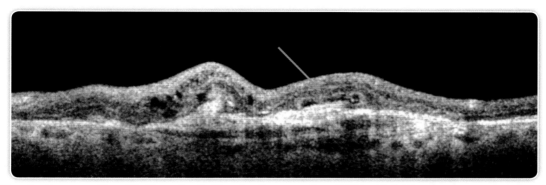

Figure 10B: Macular Degeneration. Disciform Senile Macular Degeneration OCT. In this OCT, we see serous elevation of the pigment epithelium, serous detachment of the retina, subepithelial and subretinal hemorrhages, cystoid macular edema, outer retinal tubulation (rosette appearance) (arrow). The hemorrhages infiltrate retina. Pigment deposits are always found.

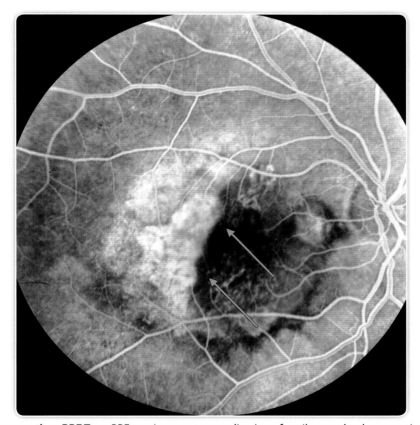

Figure 11A: Macular Degeneration. RPE Tear. RPE tear is a severe complication of senile macular degeneration. It appears in the natural evolution of serous detachment of the pigment epithelium and heavily worsens its prognosis; it is also reported to be a complication of the treatments. Tears and rips form as a result of the rupture of the pigment epithelium on the side of the serous detachment that is more distant from the fovea, on the margin between elevated epithelium and healthy epithelium.

Fluorescein angiography shows the area where RPE is removed hyperfluorescent by window defect. Normal choroidal fluorescence is seen through the opening in the pigment epithelium. The pigment epithelium flap that is free in the subretinal space can behave in two following ways: it may roll up on itself or retract. The area where RPE rolled as a papyrus is very dark (arrows), blocking the posterior layers' fluorescence.

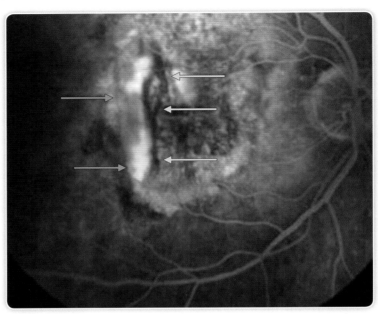

Figure 11B: Macular Degeneration. RPE Tear. The tear remain gaping in the subretinal space and RPE retracts. Fluorescein angiography shows that the area where RPE is removed is hyperfluorescent (arrows). Normal choroidal fluorescence is seen through the opening in the pigment epithelium. Here pigment epithelium flap that is free in the subretinal space retracted. The area of RPE retraction is very dark, blocking the posterior layers fluorescence (yellow arrows). The hyperfluorescent granulous micro dots correspond to an occult membrane.

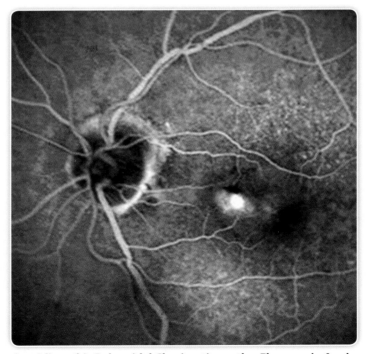

Figure 12A: Macular Degeneration. Idiopathic Polypoidal Chorioretinopathy. Fluorescein Angiography. Ophthalmoscopy shows orange colored nodules. In this fluorescein angiography, we can see a serous hemorrhagic pigment epithelium detachment intensely hyperfluorescent. Close to the optic disc is located a vascular net under the pigment epithelium linking the polypoidal angiomatous formations.

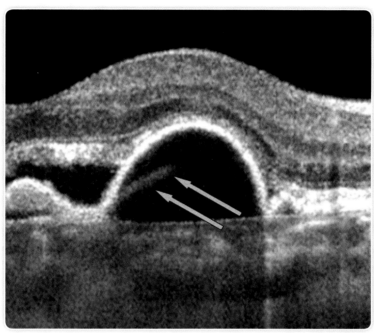

Figure 12C: Macular Degeneration. Idiopathic Polypoidal Chorioretinopathy. Cross Section OCT. This figure shows a vascular membrane under the pigment epithelium detachment and a vascular stalk (arrows) linking the choriocapillaris to the polypoidal angiomatous formation.

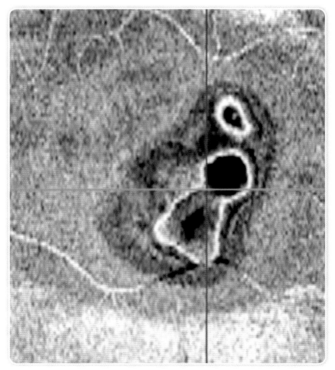

Figure 12D: Macular Degeneration. Idiopathic Polypoidal Chorioretinopathy. "En Face" OCT. The en face OCT section at the cupola cuts through the polypoidal angiomatous formation.

OTHER MACULAR DEGENERATIONS

MACULAR PATTERN DYSTROPHY

Pattern dystrophy is a frequent maculopathy that shows pattern degeneration with star-shaped dark lines. Pigment deposits in the retina form a screen against the normal fluorescence of the choroid. Blocking is total. It can be a simple pattern or a more complex pattern degeneration with a net of typically branching pigmented lines. Pigment deposits in the retina block the normal fluorescence of the choroid. In Fundus Auto Fluorescence images, pigment deposits are irregularly fluorescent. They show a pattern image with typically branching hyperfluorescent line where fluorescein angiography showed dark pigmented lines (Figs 13 to 15).

CONGENITAL OR HEREDITARY MACULOPATHIES BULL'S EYE DYSTROPHIES

Stargardt Disease—Fundus Flavimaculatus

Stargardt disease is a juvenile-onset macular dystrophy associated with rapid central visual impairment, progressive bilateral atrophy of the foveal retinal pigment epithelium, and the frequent appearance of yellowish flecks around the macula and/or in the central and near-peripheral areas of the retina. It is an autosomal recessive genetic condition observed during the first or second decade of life. Vision is impaired. Fundus shows mottling at the fovea. Later an oval lesion about 1–2 disc diameters in size, develops at the macula, generally surrounded by yellow-white flecks. Fluorescein angiography shows a dark choroid effect found in 90% of the cases. The choroid fluorescence is masked by deposits in RPE cells. Progressively numerous dots develop hyperfluorescence due to window effect. In most of the cases, a bull's eye aspect appears. Multiple specks are seen in the posterior pole. As the disease progresses the macular lesion becomes

Table 1: Macular atrophies and dystrophies
Acquired Macular Atrophies and Dystrophies
Atrophic macular degeneration
Age-related macular degeneration
Chronic epitheliopathy
Pattern dystrophy
Drusen
Hereditary Macular Atrophies and Dystrophies
Stargardt disease
Fundus flavimaculatus
Albipunctate dystrophy
Dominant progressive foveal dystrophy (dominant Stargardt disease)
Cone dystrophy
Cone-Rod dystrophy
Central retinitis pigmentosa (inverse pigmentary dystrophy)
Pseudo-vitelliform dystrophy (Best)
Dominant hereditary drusen
Doyne honeycomb degeneration,
Hutchinson-Tay disease
Malattia leventinese
Reticular dystrophy (Sjögren)
Inflammatory Lesions
Serpiginous retinopathy
Rubella syndrome
Acute posterior multifocal placoid pigment epitheliopathy
Toxoplasmosis
Toxic
Chloroquine
Phenothiazine
Ethambutol
Indomethacin
Griseofulvin
Tamoxiphen

more extensive. Atrophic changes appear in the pigment epithelium and lesions in the photoreceptors. The final visual acuity is generally 20/200. A neovascular membrane may develop.

In bull's eye macular dystrophy, fluorescein angiography shows generally two hyperfluorescent rings surrounding a dark spot. Progressively numerous dots develop an hyperfluorescence due to window effect. CNV is a rare but possible complication.

Bull's eye maculopathy is a syndrome that can have many diverse etiologies (Figs 16 to 18).

It can be **hereditary as in** Stargardt disease, Cone dystrophy, Rod cone dystrophy, or rare hereditary disorders as in benign concentric annular dystrophy, Laurence Moon Bardet Biedl syndrome. **Fundus flavimaculatus** is a condition similar to Stargardt disease with a central bull's eye lesion, but yellow flecks are more prominent and irregular in size, scattered throughout the posterior poles of both eyes, frequently extending to the equator. **Cone-Rod dystrophy is an** autosomal recessive cone-rod dystrophy that causes deterioration of the cone rod photoreceptor cells and often results in blindness. Genetic variations in the ABCA4 gene have been associated with several retinal phenotypes, including Stargardt Disease and cone-rod dystrophy.

Bull's eye maculopathy could be secondary to intoxication by Chloroquine, Hydroxychloroquine or Tamoxiphen.

Table 2: Hereditary macular dystrophies
Frequent
Stargardt disease
Fundus flavimaculatus
Albipunctate dystrophy
Cone rod dystrophy
Central retinitis pigmentosa (inverse pigmentary dystrophy)
Pseudo Vitelliform dystrophy (Best)
Dominant hereditary drusen
Rare
Doyne honeycomb degeneration
Hutchinson-Tay disease
Malattia leventinese
Reticular dystrophy (Sjögren)

Table 3: Bull's eye maculopathy
Hereditary
Stargardt disease
Cone dystrophy
Rod cone dystrophy
Benign concentric annular dystrophy
Laurence Moon Bardet Biedl syndrome
Hereditary ataxia
Batten disease
Toxic
Chloroquine dystrophy
Hydroxychloroquine dystrophy
Tamoxiphen

Table 4: Causes of retinal scars
Advanced macular degeneration
Diabetic fibrovascular membrane
Laser scars
Toxoplasmosis, multifocal choroiditis
Chorioretinitis
Trauma

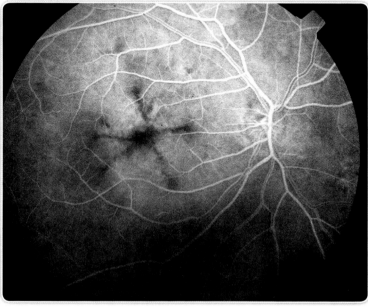

Figure 13: Macular Degeneration. Pattern Dystrophy Fluorescein Angiography. This fluorescein angiography shows pattern degeneration with star-shaped dark lines. Pigment deposits in the retina form a screen against the normal fluorescence of the choroid. Blocking screen is total.

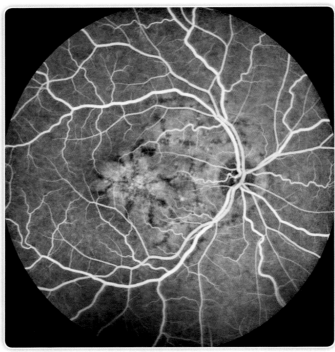

Figure 14: Macular Degeneration. Pattern Dystrophy Fluorescein Angiography. In this figure we see a complex pattern degeneration with a wide net of typically branching pigmented lines. Pigment deposits in the retina block the normal fluorescence of the choroid.

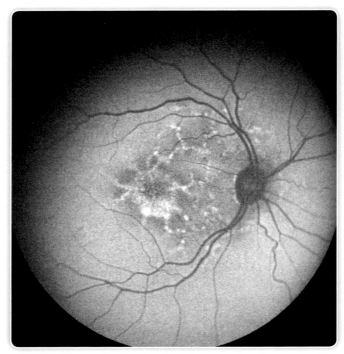

Figure 15: Macular Degeneration. Pattern Dystrophy Fundus Autofluorescence. Same case. Pigment deposits in the retina in the fundus autofluorescence images are irregularly fluorescent. In this figure, we see a macular pattern degeneration with typically branching hyperfluorescent line where fluorescein angiography showed dark pigmented lines.

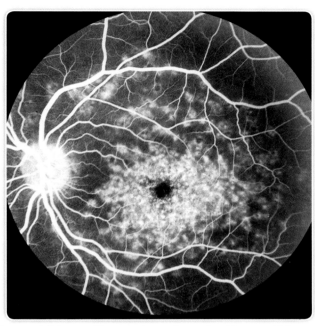

Figure 16: Macular Degeneration. Stargardt Disease. Fluorescein angiography. 18-year-old Stargardt patient. Fluorescein angiography in Stargardt disease shows a dark choroid effect found in 90% of the cases. The choroid fluorescence is masked by dense deposits in RPE cells. Progressively numerous dots develop hyperfluorescence due to window effect. In most of the cases, a bull's eye aspect appears. Multiple specks are seen in the posterior pole, mainly inside the vascular arcade.

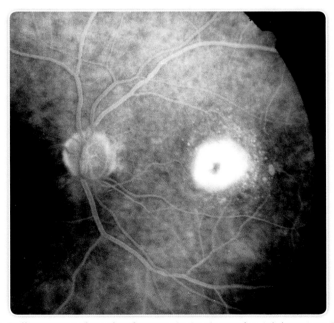

Figure 17: Macular Degeneration. Bull's Eye Maculopathy Fluorescein Angiography. Adult patient. Fluorescein angiography here does not show a dark choroid effect. In this case, the bull's eye aspect shows two hyperfluorescent rings surrounding a dark spot. Progressively numerous dots develop an hyperfluorescence due to window effect. CNV is a rare but possible complication.
Bull's eye maculopathy is a syndrome that can have many diverse etiologies. It can be **hereditary as in** Stargardt disease, Cone dystrophy, Rod-cone dystrophy, or rare hereditary disorders as in benign concentric annular dystrophy, Laurence Moon Bardet Biedl syndrome. It could be secondary to intoxication by Chloroquine, Hydroxychloroquine or Tamoxiphen.

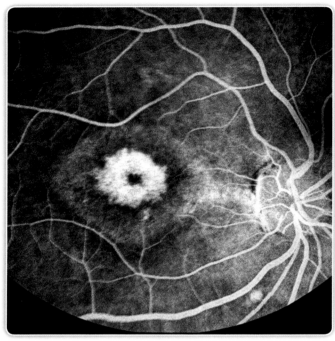

Figure 18: Macular Degeneration. Bull's Eye Maculopathy Fluorescein Angiography. The bull's eye aspect shows two hyperfluorescent rings surround a dark spot. Some hyperfluorescent dots develop, due to window effect.

Vascular Occlusions

VENOUS OCCLUSION

Venous occlusion may cause two fundamental pathologic responses: abnormalities of vascular permeability and retinal ischemia. Venous occlusions may therefore be divided into:

- *Edematous forms.* The abnormal permeability of dilated capillaries causes retinal edema, hemorrhages and exudates, and entails intraretinal leakage of the fluorescein.
- *Ischemic forms.* Ischemia occurs with the appearance of cotton-wool exudates and in the presence of extensive districts of non-perfused capillaries. Retinal hypoxia is the stimulus that causes the appearance of new vessels in the retina and iris. Unlike branch occlusions, retinal neovascularization is not very frequent in central occlusions probably because in these cases there is no vital endothelial substrate that can give rise to the new vessels proliferation.
- *Mixed forms.* The classification into edematous retinopathy and ischemic retinopathy, as a consequence of the venous occlusion process is approximate because there are many mixed forms. This is why we prefer to classify them as forms belonging mainly to one type or the other. Moreover, forms that are initially edematous may in time evolve into ischemic forms.
- *Central retinal vein (CRV) occlusions in young people.* These are generally inflammatory occlusions and regress spontaneously (Fig. 1).

EVOLUTION

CENTRAL RETINAL VEIN OCCLUSIONS

The evolution of the Central Retinal Vein occlusions varies in relation to a number of factors:

a. Factors related to age and cause of the obstruction;
b. Extent and degree of the obstruction: its site in relation to the lamina cribrosa and the anatomic possibilities for development of optical-ciliary anastomoses.
c. The fluorescein angiography is mandatory for the diagnosis and study of the evolution of venous occlusions and above all it is important to decide what treatment should be prescribed. The fluorescein angiographic examination of the entire fundus, provides a full picture of all the areas affected by the occlusion and of those that may have been spared by the process.

It also allows for an early observation of new vessels with their typical dye leakage patterns. In these cases, fluoroiridography may be also useful in that it allows to follow the onset of an rubeosis iridis that precedes vascular glaucoma.

Non-treated evolution is almost always negative except for the juvenile forms that often regress spontaneously. In the edematous capillaropathy, where stasis and capillary dilation predominate there is rapid onset of a macular edema that in time develops into cystoid macular edema with a severe and irreversible visual loss. In the forms with ischemic capillaropathy where capillary non-perfusion predominates and arterioles are affected, new vessels may appear, with severe danger of hemorrhages.

In many cases, non-perfusion leads to vascular glaucoma (Figs 2 and 3).

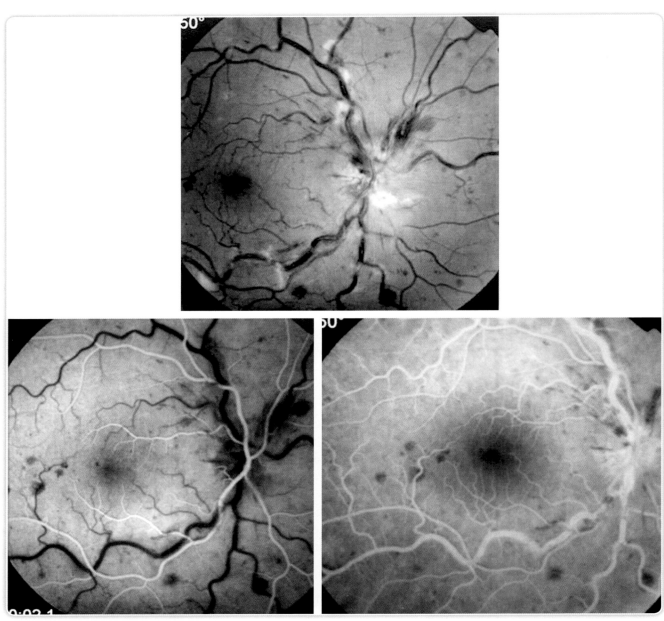

Figure 1: Vascular Occlusion. Central Venous Occlusion in Young. Patient Early to Late Fluorescein Angiography. Vein dilatation is seen with wall staining. Blood flow is slow. Venous filling is late. Hemorrhages are scattered. They can be flame shaped or rounded. Some degree of papilledema is seen. These occlusions generally regress spontaneously.

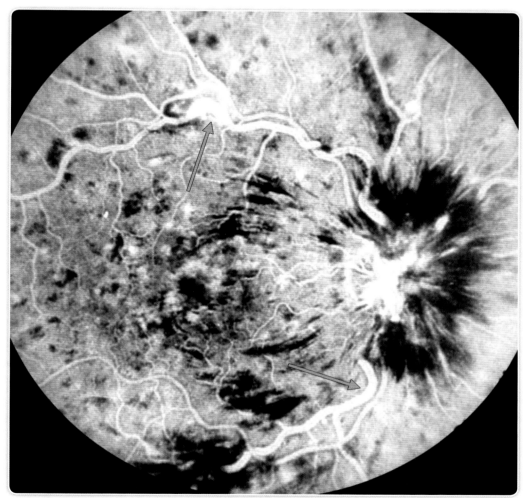

Figure 2: Vascular Occlusion. Edematous Occlusion of the Central Vein of the Retina. Venous obstruction may cause two fundamental responses: anomalies of vascular permeability and retinal ischemia. The case shown is an edematous case. The anomalous permeability of dilated capillaries causes retinal edema, hemorrhages and exudates, and entails intraretinal leakage of the fluorescein.
Fluorescein angiography is necessary for the diagnosis and study of the evolution of venous occlusions and above all it is indispensable to decide whether, when, and what treatment should be prescribed. The fluorescein angiographic examination of the entire fundus, provides a full picture of all the areas affected by the occlusion and of those that may have been spared by the process. There is edema of the retina and of the optic disc. Veins are enlarged with irregular vascular dilations (arrows). Hemorrhages can be seen in all retina, flame shaped or radial along nerve fibers when superficial, rounded when located in the deeper retinal layers.

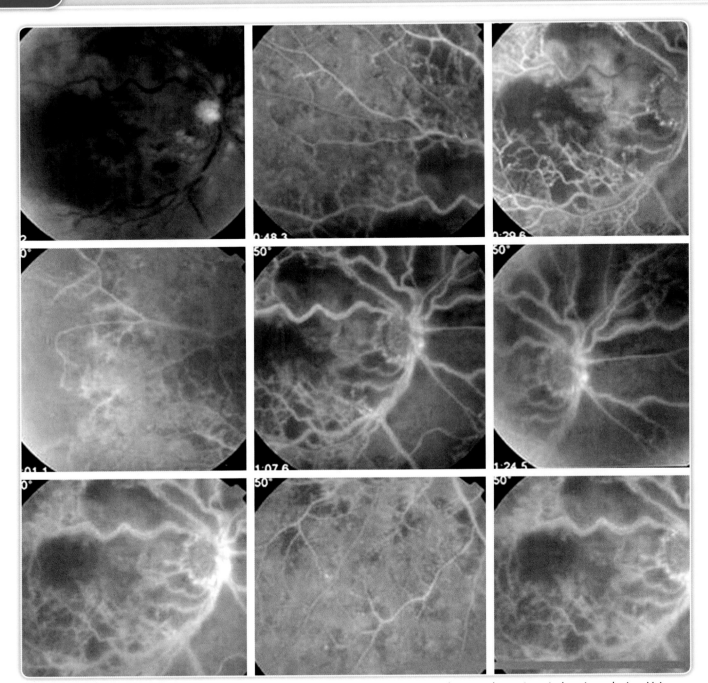

Figure 3: Vascular Occlusion. Ischemic Occlusion of the Central Vein of the Retina. The case shown is an ischemic occlusion. Veins are enlarged with irregular dilatations. Hemorrhages can be seen in all retina, flame shaped or radial along nerve fibers when superficial, rounded when in the deeper retinal layers. Non-perfused areas are seen mainly around the optic disc and in nasal retina. Non-perfused retina is darker than normally perfused retina. Frequently ischemic non-treated occlusions evolve toward vascular glaucoma.

RETINAL VEIN BRANCH OCCLUSION

The venous branch occlusions may be divided into ischemic, edematous or mixed forms depending on the alterations described earlier, located in this case in smaller retinal districts. It is important to locate the site of the occlusion through fluorescein angiography. The occlusion seat is generally located at an arteriovenous crossing and the wall of the vein involved is brightly stained with dye. There may also be leakage of fluorescein. In the branch venous occlusion, area the capillaries are clearly dilated and tortuous and there is leakage. Often hemorrhages and exudates cover the whole district involved. When the macular capillary network is affected visual loss occurs at an early stage.

In the edematous forms, at the periphery of the affected area, collateral circulation may appear with venous and also arteriovenous anastomoses formed by dilated capillaries. An interruption in the perifoveal arcade is a negative prognostic sign for visual function. At the level of some anastomosis vessel, the veins may be reopen with retrograde flow (Figs 4 to 7).

In the ischemic or mixed forms of venous branch occlusions, new vessels may appear on the edges of the area involved. In these cases, localized laser treatment is required in the areas of non-perfusion to avoid the onset of hemorrhages and, in some cases, of vascular glaucoma.

Table 1: Causes of venous occlusion

Venous occlusions are caused by three factors: alterations in vessel wall; hemodynamic disorders, blood disease. We subdivide the causes according to frequency:

Frequent causes
Retinal arteriosclerosis
Diabetic retinopathy
Hypertension

Blood disorders
Leukemia
Polyglobulemia
Diglobulemia
Polycythemia
Anemias
Sickle cell anemia
Thalassemia
Anticardiolipin
Contraceptive hormonal treatment

Less frequent causes
Vasculitis
Eales' disease
Focal infections

Ocular frequent causes
Retinal thrombophlebitis
Glaucoma
Ocular trauma
Vein malformations
Hippel Lindau
Drusen of the optic disc
Vasculitis
Radiation retinopathy

Systemic rare causes
Hyperviscosity syndromes
Cryoglobulinemia
Macroglobulinemia
Leukemia
Lupus erythematosus
Other blood diseases
Takayasu syndrome
Endocarditis
Harada's disease
Behçet's disease

Infection
Bacterial infections
Rickettsia
Brucellosis
Viral infections
Herpes Zoster
Influenza
Epstein Barr
Hemorrhagic fevers

Regional rare causes
Cavernous sinus thrombosis
Carotid artery occlusion
Intra or retro-ocular compression (meningioma, etc.)
Optic nerve tumors
Orbit tumors

Table 2: Causes of retinal arterial occlusion

Emboli	Other internal carotid diseases
Cardiac lesions	Temporal arteritis
Mitral valve lesions	Polyarteritis nodosa
Artificial cardiac valves	Oral contraceptives
Endocarditis	Migraine
Aortic aneurysms	Scleroderma
Cardiac catheterization	Orbital cellulitis
Arteriography and other diagnostic procedures	Wegener granulomatosis
Talcum in self-injected drugs	Dermatomyositis
Fat emboli in open bone fracture	Takayasu syndrome
Purtscher syndrome	
	Ocular high pressure
Vascular obliteration	Angle closure glaucoma
Hypertension	Ocular trauma
Atheroma of the carotid artery	Accidental ocular high pressure during surgical procedure

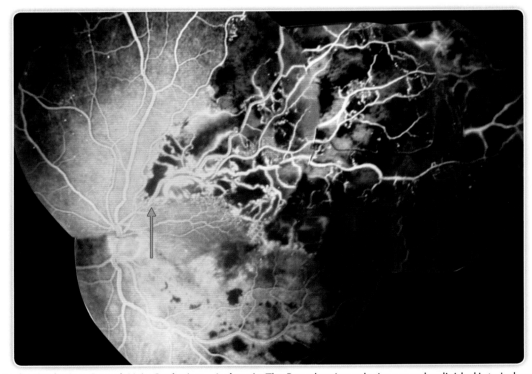

Figure 4A: Vascular Occlusion. Branch Vein Occlusion—Ischemic. The Branch vein occlusions may be divided into ischemic, edematous or mixed occlusions depending on the alterations described in the text. It is important to locate the site of the occlusion. The case illustrated here is an ischemic branch occlusion. The occlusion is located at an arteriovenous crossing (arrow) and the vein wall involved is brightly stained with dye. Veins are enlarged with irregular dilatations and stained by fluorescein. Hemorrhages are flame shaped or radial along nerve fibers when superficial, rounded when in the deeper retinal layers. Non-perfused gray areas are seen in the affected retina.

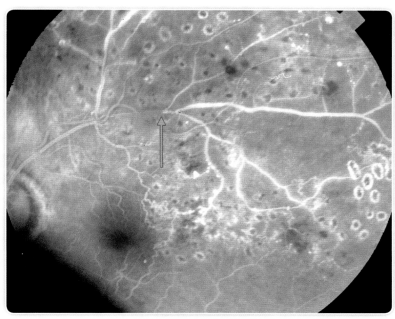

Figure 4B: Vascular Occlusion. Branch Vein Occlusion—Ischemic. The figure shows an ischemic branch occlusion. The occlusion is, as always, located at an arteriovenous crossing (arrow). The vein wall involved is stained with dye. Veins show irregular dilatations and arteriovenous shunts. Hemorrhages are rounded, located in the deeper retinal layers. We observe large non-perfused areas and some laser scars. Laser treatment needs to be completed.

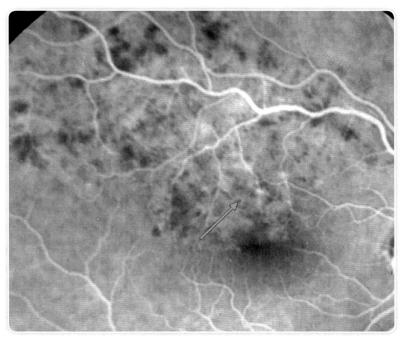

Figure 5: Vascular Occlusion. Edematous Branch Vein Occlusion. In this edematous branch vein occlusion, we can see diffuse edema and hemorrhages. At the periphery of the affected area, collateral circulation may appear with venous and also arteriovenous anastomoses formed by dilatated capillaries at the periphery. An interruption in the peri-foveal arcade is a negative prognostic sign for visual function (arrow).

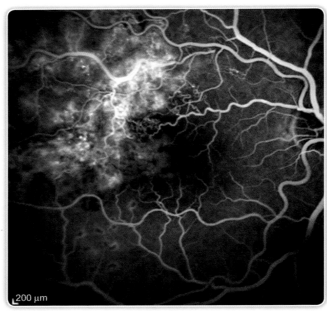

Figure 6: Vascular Occlusion. Branch Vein Occlusion—Ischemic Edematous (Mixed Form). In the area of branch venous occlusion the capillaries are clearly dilated and tortuous and there is leakage. Non-perfused areas are seen in the affected retina. Some hemorrhages and exudates cover the districts involved. When the macular capillary network is affected visual loss occurs at an early stage.

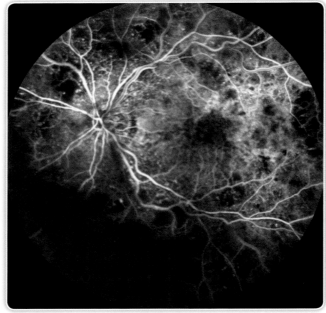

Figure 7: Vascular Occlusion. Branch Vein Occlusion—Ischemic Edematous (Mixed Form). Capillaries clearly dilated and tortuous and there is leakage. One vein segment is strongly stained by the dye. Some hemorrhages and exudates cover the districts involved. The macular capillary network is affected. Non-perfused areas and edematous areas are seen in the affected district.

In mixed venous branch occlusions, new formed vessels may appear on the edges of the area involved. In these cases, localized photocoagulation treatment is required in the areas of non-perfusion to avoid the onset of hemorrhages and, in some cases, of vascular glaucoma.

ARTERY OCCLUSION

CENTRAL RETINAL ARTERIAL OCCLUSION

Fluorescein angiography of occlusion of the central retinal artery shows non-perfusion of the arteries and frequently of the venous vascular network. It can show sometimes some edema .

The OCT performed in the first few days of a an occlusion of the central retinal artery shows retinal edema, *localized in the inner layers*: the nerve fiber layer, the ganglion cell layer, the inner plexiform layer and the layer of the bipolar cells. An increase in the reflectivity and thickness of the inner nuclear layer and the nerve fiber layer can be observed.

After a few months, *an atrophy of the inner retina* can be seen, with disruption and thinning of the inner retinal layers (Figs 8 and 9)

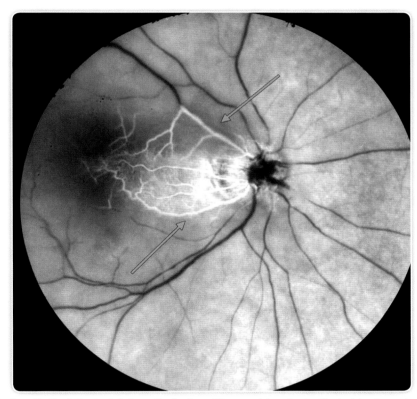

Figure 8: Vascular Occlusion. Retinal Central Artery Occlusion. 60-year-old patient affected by hypertension. Black non-perfused arteries and grey non-perfused areas are seen in the affected retina. Only a small district involving a ciliary artery has been spared and is normally perfused (arrows).

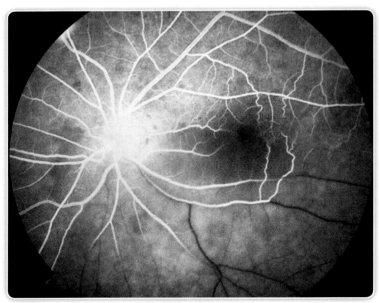

Figure 9: Vascular Occlusion. Branch Artery Occlusion. In this case of branch artery **occlusion,** we see absence of filling of some artery segments and of the vascular district involved. Filling however occurs at the later phases, very slowly or through retrograde flow. One branch of the artery is occluded. Most retina has been spared and is normally perfused. Non-perfused arteries and non-perfused areas can seen in the affected retina on the temporal inferior side.

Retinal Epitheliopathies

CENTRAL SEROUS CHORIORETINOPATHY

Central serous chorioretinopathy usually occurs in men between 25 and 45 years of age; it is often bilateral and recurrent.

Fluorescein angiography reveals one or many leakage points that appear early and increase progressively in size and fluorescence. In serous pigment epithelium detachments, the dye pools where the pigment epithelium is detached from Bruch's membrane, forming bubbles that fill with fluorescein dye.

The OCT shows importance and extent of the serous retinal detachment, the importance, localization and number of the pigment epithelium detachments. It sometimes shows a small break in the pigment epithelium at the place where a leakage is seen on fluorescein angiography. From this break, we may occasionally see fibrin that seems to leak from the choroid toward the interior of the detachment. At the level of serous detachment inner limit, we can see that the IS/OS junction (ellipsoid) and the tips of the photoreceptors are elevated, showing a marked reflectivity. In most eyes with active serous chorioretinopathy, after a few weeks evolution, we can see alteration of the outer segment of the photoreceptors. The outer photoreceptor segment may be thickened, irregular or have increased reflectivity, with granulations or flaking of the internal face of the detachment in the detached area (Figs 1A and B).

CHRONIC EPITHELIOPATHY OR DIFFUSE RETINAL PIGMENT EPITHELIOPATHY

Chronic epitheliopathy usually occurs in patients 45 to 69 years of age. Fluorescein angiography shows leakage, dystrophic changes of the pigment epithelium and serous pigment epithelium detachments. Areas of the pigment epithelium may be absent, and areas of gravitational epitheliopathy can be observed. Choroidal neovascularization is common.

In the advanced, chronic form of serous chorioretinopathy, with partial resolution of the detachments, there is thinning of the outer nuclear layer associated with changes at the IS/OS junction (ellipsoid) at the OCT imaging.

Over the course of the natural history, neovascular membranes and gravitational epitheliopathies may appear.

Gravitational Epitheliopathies

In some disorders in which there is a chronic failure of the pigment epithelium with serous retinal elevation there may be vertically-arranged degenerative pillar-like or drop-shaped alterations of the pigment epithelium appearing between the original lesions and the lower retinal portion.

Fluorescein angiography reveals a more or less wide strip with well-defined boundaries that widens towards the lower part of the retina.

We may frequently observe the lesion that is at the origin of the epitheliopathy, generally a leakage. This dye leakage is located in the posterior pole or close to the optic disc. The serous elevation of the neuroepithelium progresses slowly under gravity forces towards inferior retina. The sub-retinal fluid is reabsorbed continuously by the pigment epithelium until exhaustion and degeneration of the latter. The evolution takes from a few weeks to more than a year. When the fluid reaches the retinal periphery it widens to form a drop and the ensuing atrophy of the pigment epithelium takes on a similar shape (Figs 2 to 4).

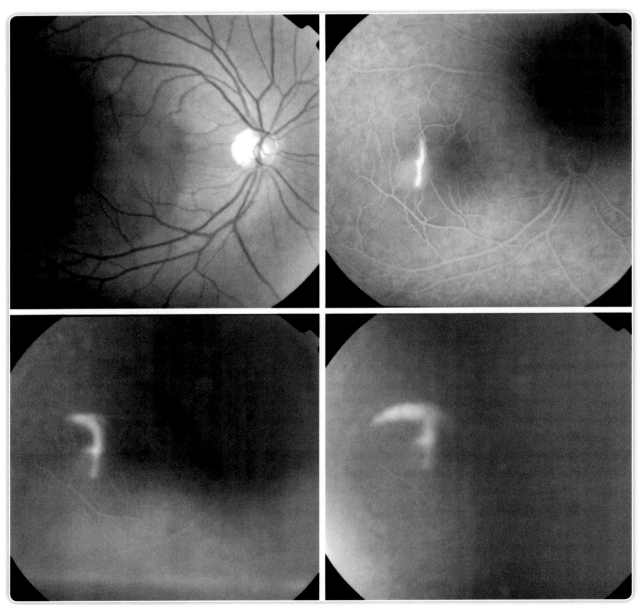

Figure 1A: Central Serous Chorioretinopathy Fluorescein Angiography. Retinal Leakage. Typical aspect of a "pine-tree" like leakage due to the diffusion of the dye in the fluid of the retinal elevation bubble. The dye reaches the bubble superior limits, and then follows the detachment limits flowing first laterally and then down.

Table 1: Causes of gravitational epitheliopathies

- Chronic central serous chorioretinopathy
- Serous- hemorrhagic disciform maculopathy
- Nevi
- Hemangioma and other tumors of the choroid
- Coloboma of the optic disc
- Optic pit
- Rare or exceptional causes

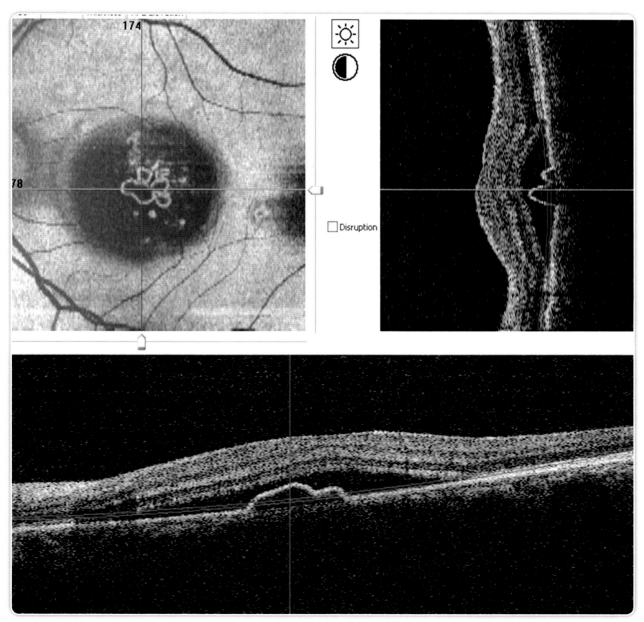

Figure 1B: Central Serous Chorioretinopathy. Cross Section and "En Face" OCT. Cross section OCT shows the pigment epithelium detachments under the retinal elevation. The "en face" OCT highlights the frontal appearance of the pigment epithelium detachments under the retinal elevation. It shows a cluster of PED when in the cross section scan there seemed to be a single detachment.

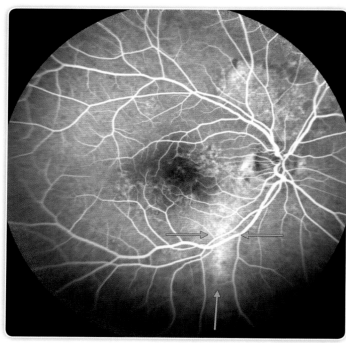

Figure 2A: Chronic Central Serous Chorioretinopathy with Gravitational Epitheliopathy Fluorescein Angiography. When there is a chronic failure of the pigment epithelium with serous retinal detachment, we can see vertical degenerative pillar-shaped alterations of the pigment epithelium between the original lesions and the lower portion. Fluorescein angiography reveals a more or less wide vertical strip of epithelium dystrophy with well-defined boundaries that widens to drop shape with atrophy of the pigment epithelium (arrows).

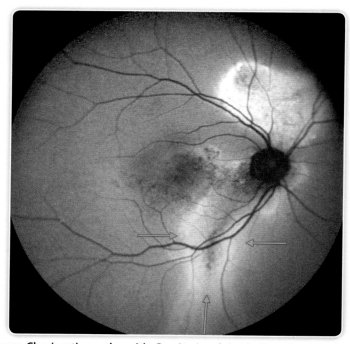

Figure 2B: Chronic Central Serous Chorioretinopathy with Gravitational Epitheliopathy (Fundus Autofluorescence Image). The hyperfluorescent lesions show that there is abnormal lipofuscin waste accumulation that cannot be absorbed by the epithelial cell. Lipofuscin is highly hyperautofluorescent. The atrophic lesions (cell apoptosis) appear as dark, hypofluorescent areas. Autofluorescence image shows a wide vertical strip of epithelium dystrophy with well-defined boundaries that widens below to drop shape (arrows).

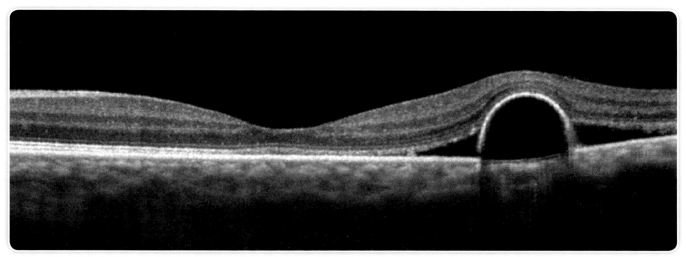

Figure 2C: Chronic Central Serous Chorioretinopathy with Gravitational Epitheliopathy, OCT. Cross section OCT shows one shallow pigment epithelium detachment and two retinal elevations with alterations of the elevated photoreceptors outer segments. The retinal pigment epithelium is atrophic in some places and we observe lesions of the junction IS/OS (ellipsoid).

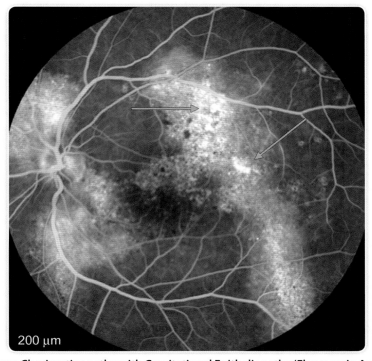

Figure 3. Chronic Central Serous Chorioretinopathy with Gravitational Epitheliopathy (Fluorescein Angiography). Serous fluid flows from some leaking lesions (arrows) elevating the retina. The pigment epithelium between the original lesions and the lower part of the retina shows dystrophic lesions. Fluorescein angiography reveals a vertical strip of epithelium dystrophy with well-defined boundaries that widens towards the lower part of the retina.

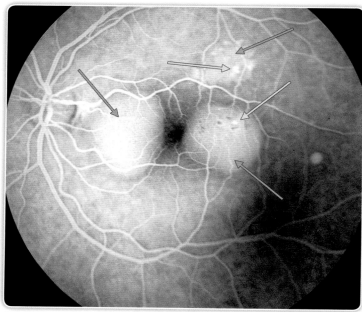

Figure 4: Central Serous Chorioretinopathy Secondary to Corticoid Treatment in Patient Operated of Kidney Transplant. Fluorescein angiography reveals in this 40 years old man operated of kidney transplant, treated by corticoids for more than 6 months, three serous retinal detachments (arrows) at the posterior pole. Three leakage points can be observed inside two of the serous retinal detachments (yellow arrows).

CHAPTER 14

Vitreoretinal Interface Syndrome

The vitreoretinal interface syndromes is caused by a glial proliferation that causes a tangential traction on its inner retinal layers; it is often observed in patients over the age of 50. These patients generally ask an eye examination when they note metamorphopsy and for visual loss, which is initially mild.

Synonyms: retraction of the internal limiting membrane, preretinal glial proliferation, epiretinal membrane, cellophane maculopathy, macular pucker.

Preretinal and Epiretinal Membrane

Epiretinal membrane can apply traction to the retinal surface, with retinal outline deformation. Vitreoretinal traction is exerted by preretinal membranes to the retinal surface, deforming its outline and sometimes inducing intraretinal fissures and cavities between elevated retinal inner layers. The traction can be antero-posterior or tangential. In the first case, we see elevations of the inner retinal layers, that can take a peaked shape. In tangential traction, retinal folds appear that may be parallel or radial. A large preretinal membrane consisting of glial tissue adhering to the retinal surface anchored to the vascular arcades contracts thus causing retinal folds. The retraction of this membrane causes retinal folds that modify the vessels path that will appear to be stretched and elongated when they are parallel to the folds, and tortuous when they cross them. Since the tractions are perpendicular to the vascular arcades they bring them closer to each other. The folds are generally transversal in the retina underlying the retracted membrane, and radial outside the retraction area. The capillaries involved show a slight leakage with staining of the retinal tissue in the later phases.

At OCT examination, the detached posterior hyaloid appears as reflective line thin but well delineated, sometimes adhering at several points to the retinal surface, which may be raised by vitreal tractions.

The preretinal membranes are usually very thin, corresponding sometimes to the detached posterior hyaloid membrane, or they can be thickened by fibroglial elements, and are very hyperreflective.

Macular Pucker

In macular pucker retinal surface irregularities are more important. Inner retina is thickened and distorted by numerous folds. Epiretinal membranes are thicker and can merge with the nerve fiber layer. Dense fibroglial tissue may appear. Frontal en face scans are important in this superficial retinal pathology showing the folds aspect and topography.

Cystoid macular edema in vitreomacular traction. The traction forces from the vitreous lead to cystoid edema formation seen as large, hyporeflective, rounded spaces in the fovea. Some irregular cells of cystoid edema are also seen below the retinal surface and in the inner and outer nuclear layers. In some cases, a real cystoid edema may appear with loggias arranged in the form of flower petals where the dye pools in the later phases.

Table 1: Causes of epiretinal membranes
• Idiopathic
• Diabetic retinopathy,
Venous occlusions
• Trauma
• Ocular surgery
• Macular degeneration
• Retinal scars
• Uveitis Choroiditis Perforating ocular wounds
After retinal detachment surgery, or as a sequel to:
• Cryoapplications
• Vitrectomy
• Laser photocoagulation

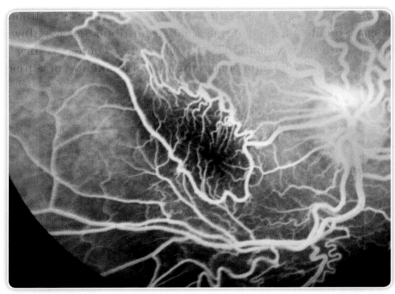

Figure 1: Vitreoretinal Interface Syndrome. Fluorescein angiography highlights morphological alterations. Retinal surface irregularities are evident. Retinal retraction modify the vessels path that appear deformed, stretched and elongated.

Diagnosis of a Dark Area in the Fluorescein Angiography

When the observation of the retina with the ophthalmoscope shows up a dark spot, apparently deep and located in the choroid, the differential diagnosis takes into account four main possibilities:

- **Deep choroidal subretinal hemorrhage that** raises the pigment epithelium and the retina forming a flat detachment. The blood may infiltrate the retina and appear at its surface, the edges are sharp, and in fluorescein angiography, it forms a full screen.
- **Epithelial hypertrophy** corresponds to a thickening of the pigment epithelium. At this point, the cells are hyperpigmented and larger in size. At the site of the alteration the retina is flat, not elevated, the retinal vessels normally pass over the dark spot that presents very sharp borders and some dots of irregular hyperfluorescence (Figs 2 to 4).
- **In the nevus of the choroid** the retina is not elevated or slightly elevated (less than 1 mm), the retinal vessels pass normally in front of the dark area whose margins are sharp but less so than in the case of the pigment epithelium hypertrophy. The screen is not total (Fig. 1). The choroid is hyperpigmented. At the OCT, nevus show a highly reflective strand in the anterior choroid below pigment epithelium with dense shadow on the posterior layers that masks choroidal vessels and sclera drusen: are frequently seen. In long-standing nevi, subretinal fluid can appear. Subretinal neovascularization is a possible complication (Fig. 1).
- **In the melanoma of the choroid**, the choroid is entirely infiltrated and destroyed by the tumor elements; the normal structure disappears and in its stead are the abnormal vessels of neoformation and the intratumor hemorrhages. Bruch's membrane and the pigment epithelium are altered and tumor elements break through, crossing these structures, thus forming subretinal bulges. The retina is elevated both for the tumor and for serous fluid; subretinal and preretinal hemorrhages frequently occur (Fig. 5).

Other diagnostic possibilities are the other tumors of the choroid,

Metastatic tumors that have little pigmentation and are often multiple (Fig. 6).

Angiomas of the choroid in which fluorescein angiography reveals a marked fluorescence in the early phases.

Table 1: Diagnosis of a dark choroidal mass

OPHTHALMOSCOPY: BROWNISH OR GRAYISH ELEVATION MASS

FLUORESCEIN ANGIOGRAPHY—EARLY PHASES

Hyperfluorescence
Melanoma (irregular hyperfluorescence)
Hemangioma of the choroid
Metastatic carcinoma

Hypofluorescence due to masking
Choroidal hemorrhage
Pigment epithelium hypertrophy
Nevus of the choroid
Melanoma of the choroid

FLUORESCEIN ANGIOGRAPHY—LATE PHASES

Hyperfluorescence
Melanoma (generally irregular fluorescence)
Hemangioma of the choroid (uniform fluorescence)
Metastatic carcinoma (uniform fluorescence)

Hypofluorescence
Deep hemorrhage
Hypertrophy of the pigment epithelium
Benign nevus (hyperfluorescence of drusen, if any)

Table 2: Melanoma

Fluorescein Angiography Earliest Phase:

Deep masking, retinal vessels seem normal or dilated

Fluorescein Angiography Early Phase:

Filling of tumor vessels; the overlying retinal vessels are at times dilated and tortuous;

Hypofluorescence due to pigment, hemorrhages, poorly vascularized tumor tissue

Fluorescein Angiography Late Phase:

Generally irregular fluorescence

Dye pooling

Hyperfluorescent spots (hot spots)

Table 3: Differential diagnosis of a subretinal formation

Choroidal tumors
- **Nevus**
- **Angioma**
- **Melanoma**
- **Metastases**
- **Osteoma**

Parasitosis

Cysticercosis

Myiasis

Toxocara canis

Other formations (deposits)

Lipofuscin deposits in best disease and pseudovitelliform maculopathy

Tamoxiphen deposits

Macular atrophy (pigment or disrupted drusen material)

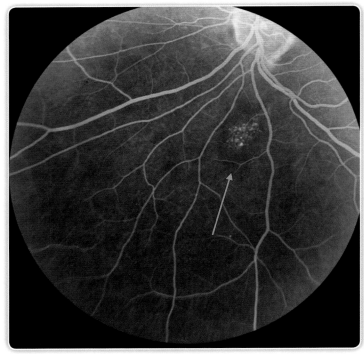

Figure 1: Dark Lesion in Fluorescein Angiography. Nevus with Drusen. Below the optic disc, we can see a dark rounded spot with some hyperfluorescent dots (arrow). The pigmented nevus formation forms a screen. Drusen are frequent and are seen as hyperfluorescent spots. In long-standing nevi, subretinal fluid can appear giving a gravitational epitheliopathy. Subretinal neovascularization is a possible complication.

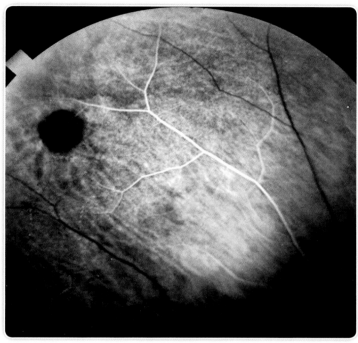

Figure 2: Dark Lesion in Fluorescein Angiography. Pigment Epithelium Hypertrophy. The pigmented formations form a dense screen, denser than nevi. Hypertrophies of the pigment epithelium are very dense, with sharp limits.

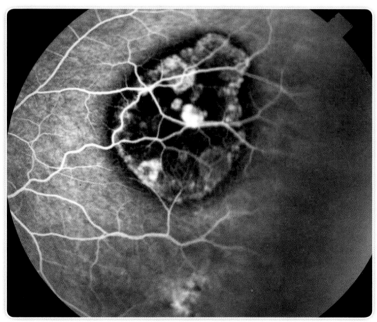

Figure 3: Dark Lesion in Fluorescein Angiography. Hyperplasia of the Pigment Epithelium. Hyperplasia of the pigment epithelium form a dense screen. They frequently are less regularly pigmented than pigment hypertrophies.

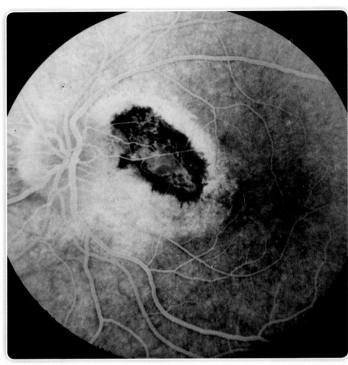

Figure 4: Dark Lesion in Fluorescein Angiography. Pigmented Scar. Some scars may be heavily pigmented as in this old toxoplasmosis choroiditis scar surrounded by RPE atrophy giving window effect hyperfluorescence.

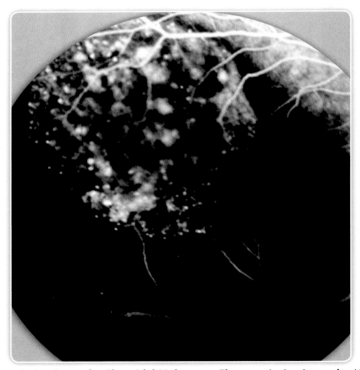

Figure 5: Dark Lesion in Fluorescein Angiography Choroidal Melanoma. Fluorescein Angiography. Under normal retinal vessels this heavily pigmented tumor mass is evident. Pooling is due to abnormal dye accumulation in the tumor mass. In the early phases of the fluoroangiography, the screen is total, and in the later stages the neoformation is irregularly fluorescent.

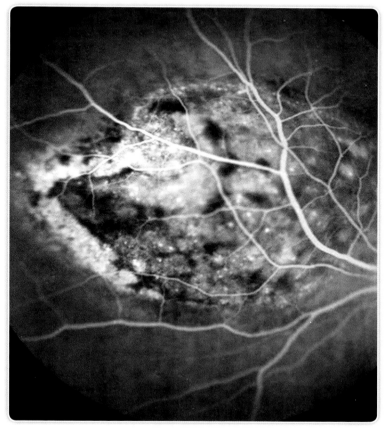

Figure 6: **Dark Lesion in Fluorescein Angiography Choroidal Metastases. Fluorescein Angiography.** Normal retinal vessels pass above this tumor mass. The neoformation is much less pigmented than in melanomas and has an irregularly rounded shape. There is some abnormal dye pooling in the mass of the tumor. The later stages show that the neoformation is irregularly fluorescent.

Inflammatory Disorders

Fluorescein angiography is an important tool, alongside OCT in the diagnosis and follow-up of ocular inflammatory disorders. Ocular inflammation leads to hyperfluorescence and hypofluorescence.

Hypofluorescence is due generally to a defect in vascular filling, more rarely due to blocked (masked) fluorescence. Vascular filling defects may be observed both in the retina and in the choroid and may be caused by artery occlusion. Frequently branch artery occlusions are seen that, at times, also show the embolus that is responsible for the obstacle to the blood flow, and in the earlier arteriovenous phases, lack of filling of the vascular district involved. Filling however may occur at the later phases, very slowly or through retrograde flow.

Capillary micro-occlusions form one have multiple causes for them and some are inflammatory. They can be seen also in inflammatory venous thrombosis, vasculitis, Eale's disease, etc.

Hyperfluorescence is due generally to leakage or pooling of the dye.

Acute choroiditis may show, as in Harada disease some multiple retinal serous detachments with intense leakage of the fluorescein. The dye then pools in the retinal detachments. This is often associated with serous elevations of the pigment epithelium and, at times, a large retinal elevation. Similar leakage cases have been described in patients with other exudative choroiditis.

SCATTERED MULTIFOCAL CHOROIDITIS AND WHITE DOTS SYNDROMES

Retinopathies that feature multiple scattered white dots (chorioretinal inflammatory localizations) form an interesting chapter of retinal inflammations. They are not uncommon in everyday practices, but there is risk of missing diagnosis as the lesions are not always easy to see.

After some mild flu-like symptoms, young adults, frequently myopic women develop an acute visual loss that varies from minimal to 20/100. Some cases are unilateral, some other bilateral. An enlargement of the blind spot is shown by visual field examination in a few patients. Most of them show some degree of posterior vitritis. Etiology remains unknown but it could be an autoimmune disease.

Fluorescein angiography shows scattered hyperfluorescent dots. ICG shows generally scattered hypofluorescent dots (Figs 1 to 4).

The OCT scans show very limited lesions in the photoreceptor layer with segmentation or interruption of the junction between inner and outer segment of the photoreceptors, that corresponds with hypofluorescent areas in the late phase of ICG. "En face" OCT scans passing exactly through the level of the junction between inner and outer segment of the photoreceptors show areas of alteration and give an exact map of the lesions.

VASCULITIS

Leakage is always seen in **vasculitis.** Sometimes, staining of the walls of the major vessels appear and then dye leakage. This leakage increases progressively in the later phases and infiltrates the surrounding retina. As usual, the edges are very blurred. A localized hyperfluorescence due to staining is noted on the vessel walls with leakage from specific points. The leaks allow the dye to penetrate into the surrounding retina, Hyperfluoresence increases in the later phases and may persist for over an hour (Figs 5 and 6).

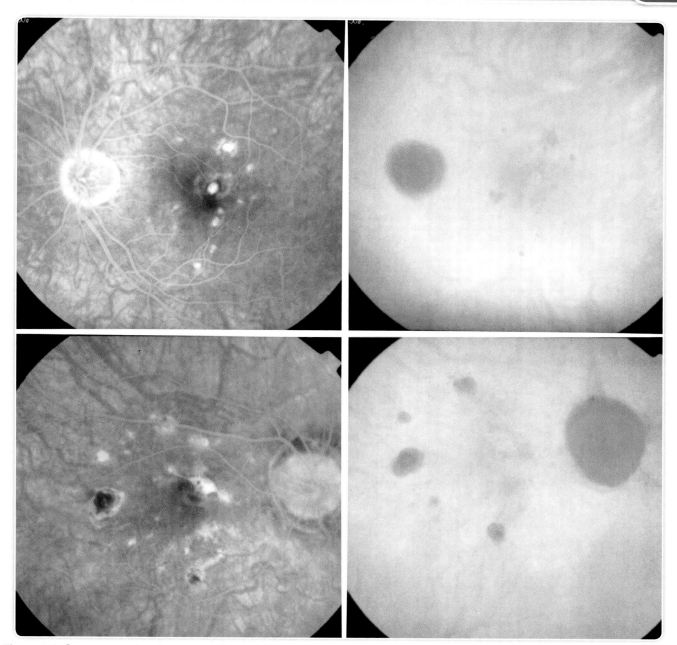

Figure 1: Inflammatory Disorders. Scattered Multifocal Choroiditis. After some mild flu-like a young (27 years old) myopic woman develops an acute bilateral visual loss. She shows some degree of posterior vitritis. Etiology remains unknown but it could be an autoimmune disease. Fluorescein angiography (left hand side) shows scattered hyperfluorescent dots. ICG shows (left hand side) scattered hypofluorescent dots.

▎FROSTED BRANCH VASCULITIS

Frosted branch vasculitis also named "angiitis", causes a retinal perivascular sheathing of both arterioles and venules in association with uveitis, retinal edema and visual loss. Retinal vasculitis is bilateral with a *'frosted' appearance.* Fluorescein angiography shows the atypical retinal perivascular sheathing of both arterioles and venules. This vasculitis can be an idiopathic disorder or can be associated with ocular and systemic diseases (Figs 7 and 8).

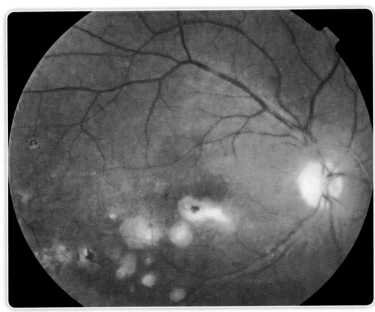

Figure 2: Inflammatory Disorders. Scattered Multifocal Choroiditis. Fundus Photograph. 30 years old myopic woman. Fundus examination reveals multiple flat white or yellowish rounded lesions scattered at the posterior pole, at level of RPE and choroid. Some lesions show pigmentation (scars).

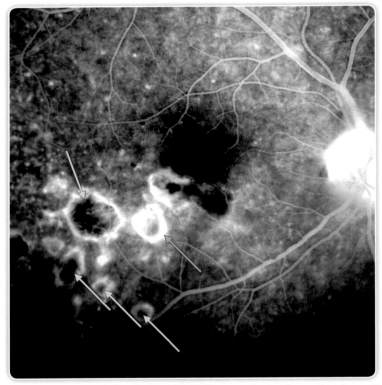

Figure 3: Inflammatory Disorders. Scattered Multifocal Choroiditis. Fluorescein Angiography. Same Case. Fluorescein angiography shows one hyperfluorescent dot with some dye leakage (active choroiditis) (arrow) close to the fovea and a dozen of scattered hypofluorescent with hyperfluorescent margins dots (scars) (yellow arrows). The optic disc is hyperfluorescent with slightly blurred margins (mild papillitis).

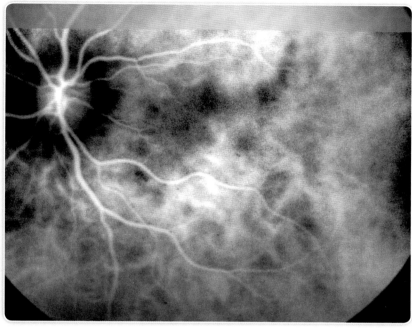

Figure 4: Inflammatory Disorders. White Dots Syndrome. Fluorescein angiography shows scattered hyperfluorescent and hypofluorescent areas and an hypofluorescent area around the optic disc.

Table 1: Indications for fluorescein angiography in inflammatory disorders
Retinal Vasculopathies
Macular complications
Cystoid macular edema
Macular, retinal and choroidal ischemia
Choroidal neovascularization
Epiretinal membrane
Detection of subtle retinal vasculopathy or choroidopathy
Noninfectious diseases
White dot chorioretinal inflammatory syndromes
Multiple evanescent white dot syndrome
Acute posterior multifocal placoid pigment epitheliopathy
Serpiginous choroiditis
Birdshot retinochoroidopathy
Multifocal choroiditis with panuveitis
Punctate inner choroidopathy
Diffuse subretinal fibrosis
Vogt-Koyanagi-Harada's syndrome
Behçet's disease
Infectious diseases

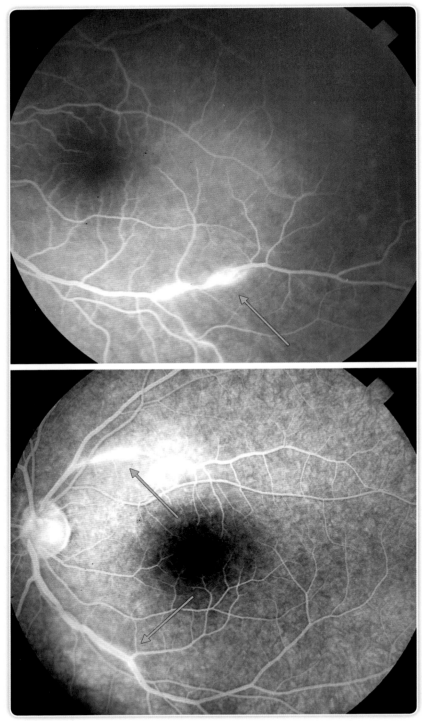

Figures 5 and 6: Inflammatory Disorders. Vasculitis. Localized hyperfluorescence of vessel segments is due to wall staining with leakage from specific points (arrows). The leakage allows the dye to penetrate into the surrounding retina, it increases in the later phases and may persist for over an hour.

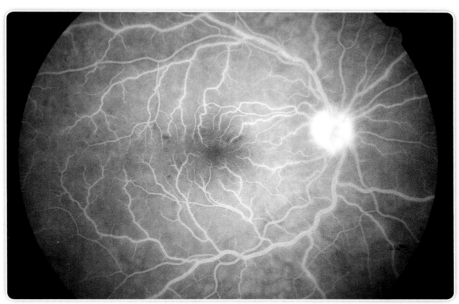

Figure 7: Inflammatory Disorders. Frosted Branch Vasculitis. Frosted branch vasculitis also named "angiitis", causes a bilateral retinal perivascular sheathing of both arterioles and venules in association with uveitis, retinal edema and visual loss. Fluorescein angiography shows the atypical retinal perivascular sheathing of both arterioles and venules with a *'frosted' appearance*.

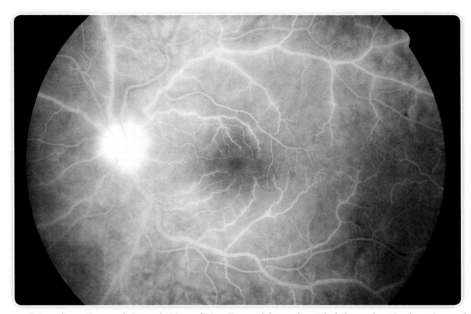

Figure 8: Inflammatory Disorders. Frosted Branch Vasculitis. Frosted branch with bilateral retinal perivascular sheathing of both arterioles and venules in association with uveitis, retinal edema and visual loss. Fluorescein angiography shows a *'frosted' branch image*.

Table 2: Infections, parasitosis causes of retinal inflammation

- Toxoplasmosis
- Cytomegalovirus
- Herpes Zoster
- Herpes simplex
- *Cryptococcus*
- Candidiasis
- Toxocara
- Cysticercosis
- Sarcoidosis
- Pars planitis
- Acute bilateral retinal necrosis

Table 3: Causes of vasculitis

Ocular diseases
Eale's disease
Uveitis
Birdshot retinopathy
Frosted branch angiitis
Idiopathic

General infections
Toxoplasmosis
Tuberculosis
Cytomegalovirus
Lyme disease
Herpes simplex
Herpes Zoster- Varicella
Brucellosis
Cat scratch disease
Other infections

Systemic diseases
Behçet disease
Sarcoidosis
Lupus erythematosus
Arteritis nodosa
Multiple sclerosis
Leukemia
Crohn's disease
Other systemic diseases

Table 4: Causes of frosted branch angiitis

Cytomegalovirus retinitis (CMV)

AIDS retinitis

Toxoplasmosis

Systemic lupus erythematosus

Crohn's disease

Large cell lymphoma and acute lymphoblastic leukemia

Focal frosted branch angiitis secondary to

Cytomegalovirus retinitis

Herpes simplex virus

Varicella zoster virus

Tuberculosis

Antistreptolysin O

Epstein-Barr virus

Coxsackie virus A10

Adenovirus

Measles

Rubella

Behçet's disease

Table 5: White dot syndromes

Bird-shot chorioretinopathy

Multiple evanescent white dot syndromes

Acute posterior multifocal placoid pigment epitheliopathy (APMPPE)

Punctate inner choroidopathy

Multifocal choroiditis

Acute retinal pigment epitheliitis or acute retinitis

Sometimes serpiginous choroiditis is associated in this group of retinal diseases

Index

Page numbers followed by *f* refer to figure and *t* refer to table